THE

COMPLETE

BOOK OF

MEDICAL SYMPTOMS

IN

CHILDREN

*

THE

COMPLETE

BOOK OF

MEDICAL SYMPTOMS

IN

CHILDREN

DR MARTIN EDWARDS

foulsham
London · New York · Toronto · Sydney

foulsham
Yeovil Road, Slough, Berkshire, SL1 4JH

ISBN 0-572-01922-X

Copyright © 1994 Dr Martin Edwards

NOTICE
In this book, the author has done his best to outline the indicated general
treatment for various childhood conditions, diseases, ailments, and their
symptoms. Also, recommendations are made regarding certain drugs,
medications and preparations.

Different people react to the same treatment, medication, or preparation in
different ways. This book does not purport to answer all questions about all
situations that you or your child may encounter. It does not attempt to
replace your physician.

Neither the author nor the publishers of this book take responsibility for
any possible consequences from any treatment, action or inaction, or
application of any medication or preparation to any child by any person
reading or following the information or advice contained in this book.
The publication of this book does not constitute the practice of medicine.
The author and publisher advise that you consult your doctor before
administering any medication or undertaking any course of treatment.

Printed in Great Britain
by St Edmunbury Press Ltd,
Bury St. Edmunds, Suffolk.

CONTENTS

INTRODUCTION

A child's illness can be sudden, worrying, confusing and – in more ways than one – messy. Illnesses don't appear as neat packages labelled 'measles' or 'appendicitis'; instead children develop a bewildering array of symptoms which you have to piece together, diagnose, and decide how best to treat.

This book aims to help you do just that. You can look up your child's symptoms and find help in working out what they mean, what you can do, and when you should see your doctor.

Why does your child cough at night? ... When is an earache serious? ... How long should you leave a vomiting child without seeking help? ... What are the symptoms that should always be checked by a doctor, whatever the time? ... These are the kind of questions that are important to parents looking after a sick child, and which this book aims to help you answer.

HOW TO USE THE BOOK

The sections of the book each cover a different main symptom, arranged alphabetically, as listed in Contents. Several diseases might be covered in each section. Overall the book provides a complete guide to childhood illnesses arranged in a way which makes it useful and easy to use. Simply turn to the section corresponding to your child's main symptom. If you are in doubt, the Index at the back of the book should help you to find the section you need.

You may like to note the following groupings. Most kinds of **pain** (for example earache, headache) are included under one of the sections covering *Pain* (using the example, in *Pain or discharge in the ear* and *Pain in the head*). **Lumps and bumps** are covered under *Lumps* (for example, *Lumps, groin or testicle, Lumps in the neck*). Similarly, **rashes and spots** are covered in *Rashes, long-term; Rashes, sudden; Spots, itchy;* and *Spots, non itchy*. Other symptoms should be in straightforward alphabetical order and simple to find.

Of course, the advice in a book such as this can only be fairly general and, if in doubt, you should SEE A DOCTOR and be guided by him or her. Most importantly, if a baby or young child simply seems very ill for whatever reason, then you should CHECK WITH A DOCTOR, regardless of whatever other symptoms are present. This advice is explained in more detail, together with a description of symptoms that should always take you to your doctor, in the section entitled *Ill – should your child see the doctor?*

As a general rule, when the book refers to a baby, a child of up to the age of 12 months is meant. A toddler means a child aged from one to about two-and-a-half years, and a schoolchild means anyone aged from five to 15 years.

SKIN COLOUR AND APPEARANCE
Several of the symptoms mentioned depend on checking the appearance of your child's skin for spots, rashes or a change in colour. In general these descriptions should apply equally well to all children but, occasionally, black children may have a slightly different appearance.

Spots or rashes which appear red in a white child, may simply produce a darkening of the skin in the same area in a black child. Fine spots, such as the rash of German measles (see *Rashes, sudden*) may be more difficult to see and may appear as slightly raised spots of normal-coloured skin. Purple spots may be slightly less difficult to see, particularly over lighter-coloured areas such as the palms and soles.

Changes in skin colour such as paleness (see *Paleness*) or jaundice, a yellow skin colour (see *Jaundice*) may be less obvious at first in black children. But even in white children the colour of the skin itself can be misleading; it is better to be guided by the colour of the membranes of the eyes or mouth (see *Paleness*) or of the whites of the eyes (see *Jaundice*). Any unusual colour of the skin itself in black children is best judged by checking the colour under the child's fingernails, or on his or her palms or soles.

DRUG DOSAGE
In several sections you will be advised to use drugs from the

chemist, and it is important to check and follow the dosage instructions that are provided with the drugs you use, according to the size and age of your child.

Paracetamol is often recommended for pain or fever; it is available as syrup, dissolvable tablets, ordinary tablets or suppositories (for rectal use – useful with vomiting children). It isn't recommended under the age of three months, although there should be no problem in using a dose of 60 milligrams (60 mg) for a two-month-old baby with a feverish reaction to vaccination (see *Immunisation reactions*).

From the age of three months to a year, a dose of 60 mg to 120 mg is recommended, and from one to six years, 120 mg to 240 mg. From six to 12 years, 250 mg to 500 mg is suitable. 500 mg is equivalent to a single ordinary adult paracetamol tablet. If you are using syrup, you must check the strength of the syrup to find how much you should give to provide the recommended dose – usually the label will tell you.

The dose can be repeated every four hours, up to a maximum of four times a day.

APPETITE

SUDDEN LOSS OF APPETITE is often a sign of illness or infection in a small baby, and should GENERALLY TAKE YOU TO YOUR DOCTOR. The same may be true for older children, although emotional upsets are often to blame, too.

POOR APPETITE OVER A LONG PERIOD may be due to a long-standing illness – possibly one that isn't obvious, such as a kidney infection or mild asthma. This is quite rare, however, and there will generally be the warning sign that the child isn't putting on weight as he or she should.

POOR APPETITE WITH NORMAL WEIGHT is far more common. Normal weight isn't the same as average weight. Some children will be considerably below average weight, and some well above, simply because of their build and height.

Your doctor or health visitor will work out whether your child is gaining weight as he or she should by plotting the weight on a centile chart (see *Weight problems*). Provided that children gain weight satisfactorily, it really doesn't matter if they are heavier or lighter than average.

❖   ❖   ❖   ❖   ❖

GUIDANCE
Feeding your child is one of the basic and most essential functions you can perform as a parent, and if your child rejects the food you provide it isn't surprising that guilt and frustration can follow. But, unfortunately, it is easy to get into mealtime patterns that can make the problem worse in the long run.

❖   ❖   ❖

Of course all children are different, and you may find that your health visitor is a good source of expert advice who can suggest just what strategy would be best for you. But these few general pointers might help.

❖   Try not to force your child to eat by spooning-in food when the child does not want it, or by threatening if he or she doesn't eat.

❖   Don't keep persuading your child to eat more, or offer bribes if he or she does.

❖   Distracting attention while you sneak in a spoonful, or 'one for teddy, one for Sammy', can store up problems in the long run.

❖   Don't let your child regularly eat snacks between meals.

❖   Don't let your child always choose what to eat at mealtimes.

Of course, all parents are guilty of some of these transgressions at some time. The problem is that, if they become established as a regular pattern of behaviour, things may never change. The child learns to be the centre of attention at meal times, and calls the tune.

❖   ❖   ❖

Very few children will allow themselves to go hungry if there is food in front of them (provided, of course, that they are old enough to feed themselves). Calmly sitting back and pretending not to care while your child eats next to nothing for days on end isn't easy, but don't be afraid to ask for help and support from your health visitor.

BED WETTING

In a class of 30 five-year-olds there are probably five or six who wet the bed at night; even a 10-year-old may be reassured that there are probably one or two others in the class who are keeping quiet about the same problem. Although dry nights virtually always appear in the end, there may be things you can do to speed them along.

THE CAUSE OF BED WETTING is very rarely a physical illness, such as a urine infection or diabetes. Your doctor can rule these out by examining a specimen of urine. Usually the cause is simply that some children take longer than others for the nerves that control their bladders to develop fully. For some reason boys are affected more often than girls.

SUDDENLY BECOMING WET AT NIGHT after being dry for some time, is often a sign of emotional stress – a new brother or sister, starting school, moving house, etc. If there is no obvious cause, then a physical illness may be to blame, and your doctor may suggest a urine test.

GUIDANCE
Your child can't help wetting the bed. Punishment, or scolding so that he or she feels ashamed or dirty, may well make things worse by increasing the child's level of stress and anxiety.

❖   ❖   ❖

Lifting small children onto the potty or toilet after they have been asleep for a few hours, will often ensure a dry bed in the morning. It saves the time, trouble and the cost of washing endless sheets, although that is all. It won't actually make the child dry any sooner.

HOME TREATMENT
It may pay you to discuss treatment with your doctor or health visitor as there are several possible strategies and it may take some trial and error to decide which is best for you.

❖   ❖   ❖

A **star chart** is often worth a try. Make a chart with a space for every day and give your child a coloured star to stick on the chart every morning that he or she is dry. A reward of a gold star or a small present after five or ten stars, gives the child something to aim for.

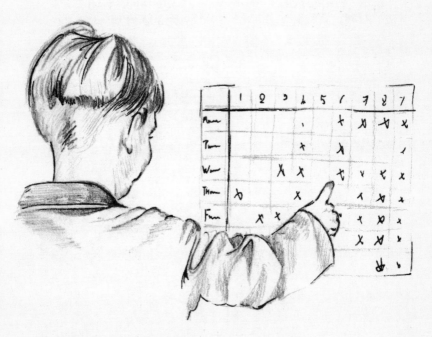

A star chart may be worth a try

✧   ✧   ✧

Some older children may do better if you give them the job of making their own beds when they are wet. Waking with a dry bed becomes a reward in itself, and the child loses any guilt or anxiety caused by making you change yet more sheets.

It is important to be sure that this isn't regarded by you or your child as a punishment for having a wet bed, but simply an opportunity for your child to be more in control of the situation.

✧   ✧   ✧

Sometimes, training children to go longer periods between weeing during the day, seems to help them become dry at night. For children aged over about seven years, alarms may help. These wake the child with a loud buzz as soon as

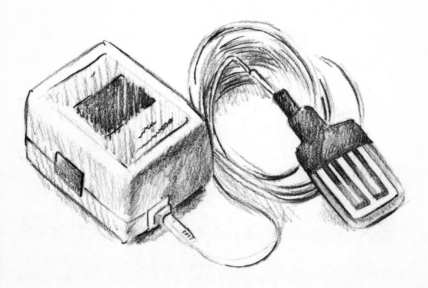

Alarms wake the child with a loud buzz as soon as the bed is wet

the bed is wetted (a sensor under the sheet detects moisture). The child learns to wake as soon as he or she begins to wee, and soon – usually within a few months – learns to wake just before.

DOCTOR'S TREATMENT
What your doctor can offer may occasionally include antidepressant drugs, which tighten the valve controlling urine flow from the bladder. **Desmopressin**, available on doctor's prescription as a nasal spray, is similar to the hormone the body produces naturally to reduce urine production. It can be dramatically effective for short periods, such as when a child goes to camp or to a friend's house, but doesn't often provide a long-term cure.

BIRTHMARKS

There are a few common types of birthmark, most of which disappear within the first few years of life.

STORK MARKS are usually obvious from birth. You will see a flat, pink, sometimes blotchy area of skin between your baby's eyebrows, in the centre of the forehead, and often on the nape of the neck. Crying makes it look worse, but the rash will fade over the next couple of years and eventually disappear. The cause is a collection of abnormal capillaries – tiny blood vessels under the skin that haven't developed properly.

The rash is called a stork mark because it is supposed to be the mark left by the stork's beak as it held your baby's head while delivering him or her across the rooftops!

A STRAWBERRY NAEVUS is also a collection of abnormal capillaries but, unlike a stork mark, it can appear almost anywhere. It appears a few days after birth, and gradually gets bigger over the first few months of life. At first it appears as a soft, raised red lump but after a few months it becomes flatter and paler with sunken white spots on the surface. At this stage it may look a little like a strawberry, hence the name strawberry naevus.

Most eventually vanish on their own, usually by the age of about seven years, and don't leave a scar or mark. Rarely, surgery may be necessary for those which won't go.

PORT WINE STAINS are the flat purple patches of skin that are familiar on many adults, because unfortunately they are permanent and won't fade. They can appear anywhere, and again are caused by abnormal capillaries.

HOME TREATMENT
Cosmetic skin camouflage creams can usually make them invisible, and the **Red Cross** offers an expert skin

camouflage service – contact your local branch for details.
DOCTOR'S TREATMENT
Nowadays, surgery by laser can give excellent results, too,
and may make the marks virtually invisible, although its
effects on children are less predictable and your doctor may
suggest waiting until your child is older.

MONGOLIAN BLUE SPOT is the name given to the blue
or grey patches of skin that sometimes appear over babies'
buttocks. They appear only in black or oriental babies, and
disappear by the age of about five years. They can look
rather like bruises, but are quite harmless.

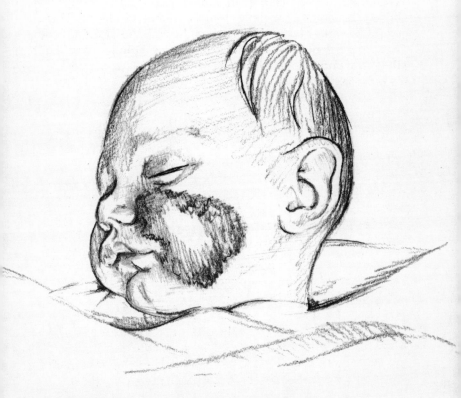

A strawberry naevus almost always disappears on its own

MOLES AND FRECKLES can appear at any time, but usually after the age of two. They are caused by an excess of melanin, the skin's brown pigment, in one spot. They are harmless but it pays to protect them from the sun because of the small risk of a mole turning cancerous. A large flat brown area of skin should be CHECKED BY A DOCTOR; it could be a **CAFE-AU-LAIT PATCH** which, although often harmless, is occasionally a sign of disease of the brain or nerves.

GUIDANCE
Watch out for any change in a mole, particularly if it grows bigger, becomes irregular or blotchy, itches, or bleeds. These could be signs of cancerous change, so SEE YOUR DOCTOR. Keep a particular eye on moles that are too big to cover with the blunt end of a pencil.

BLOOD IN THE STOOLS

Although this is alarming, and should prompt a VISIT TO YOUR DOCTOR, it may well not be a sign of anything serious.

NEWBORN BABIES sometimes swallow some of their mother's blood during birth, and pass it from the bowel soon after. Otherwise, bleeding from the rectum is rare in the first weeks of life and may be a sign of a more serious problem such as damage to the bowel or a problem with its blood supply.

OLDER BABIES AND TODDLERS quite often pass blood from the anus. Usually the cause is an **anal fissure** – a tear in the skin lining the anus – often caused by straining to pass a hard stool.

OLDER CHILDREN may suffer a fissure, too. Usually there isn't a great deal of blood, and it appears on the surface of the stool, or after it, rather than being mixed in. Opening the bowels becomes very painful, and a vicious circle may set in: the child holds on rather than having to open his or her bowels, which makes the stool even bigger and harder and the moment more painful when it finally does arrive.

DOCTOR'S TREATMENT
Usually, a fissure will heal on its own provided that you manage to keep your child's bowels quite loose. Your doctor may suggest an ointment to soothe the pain and if necessary treatment for constipation (see *Constipation*).

Occasionally an operation, to stretch the anus or remove the fissure, is necessary for the few that don't heal.

BLEEDING WITH STOMACH PAINS should always be taken seriously. There are dozens of possible causes but **intussusception**, a blockage of part of the bowel, is relatively common especially around two to six months. The child tends to scream in pain in spasms, and may be pale and quiet in between attacks. He or she may vomit, and the abdomen become blown out. This is an emergency and you should SEE YOUR DOCTOR IMMEDIATELY.

DOCTOR'S TREATMENT
An operation to relieve the blockage may well be necessary.

BLOODY DIARRHOEA is most likely to be due to an infection, often one of the food poisoning bugs such as salmonella or campylobacter. **Dysentery** is another possibility following a trip abroad. Some of these infections can make children, especially young babies, very ill. Others may seem to have little effect. SEE YOUR DOCTOR even if your child seems mildly affected.

DOCTOR'S TREATMENT
Although most of these infections get better on their own, some will respond to a course of antibiotics. The doctor is likely to be guided by your child's overall state of health in deciding on treatment, and will probably suggest a laboratory examination of your child's diarrhoea to identify the bugs responsible.

❖　　　❖　　　❖

If food poisoning bacteria are to blame, then the doctor is required, by law, to notify the local public health authorities, and you should keep your child away from friends until the infection has cleared. Usually this takes a week or two, but may occasionally take several weeks, or even longer. Other treatment is the same as for other forms of diarrhoea (see *Diarrhoea*).

NOSE BLEEDS or even a sore throat, may cause bloody stools if the child swallows enough blood.

RARER CAUSES are numerous. Stomach ulcers or inflammation can cause enough bleeding for blood to appear at the other end; polyps or abnormal blood vessels inside the bowel can cause large bleeds. **Colitis**, an inflammation of the lower part of the bowel whose cause is unknown, is more common in older children and adults; although the symptoms come and go it may well need life-long treatment. Often, after tests and examinations, doctors just can't come up with the cause of the bleeding.

❖   ❖   ❖   ❖   ❖

GUIDANCE
SEE YOUR DOCTOR if your child develops blood in his or her stool. If the blood is mixed in with the stool then SEE THE DOCTOR IMMEDIATELY, as this suggests that the bleeding is actually coming from inside the bowel. Blood on the surface of the stool suggests bleeding from the anus, probably caused by a fissure, and is less urgent.

BOILS

A boil develops when a hair follicle – the skin pore from which a hair grows – becomes infected. Usually the culprit is a bacterium called **staphylococcus aureus**, the same bacterium that is responsible for impetigo (see *Rashes, long-term*) and several other skin infections.

THE APPEARANCE OF A BOIL is familiar to most people. A tender red spot appears, and grows over the next few days. At first it feels solid; as it enlarges liquid yellow pus starts to build up in its centre. This gives the spot a white or yellow top which feels tense. A boil full of pus which is on the point of bursting is said to be pointing.

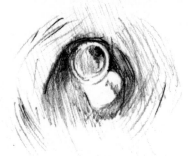

A boil passes through several different stages

Usually a boil bursts on its own, often with instant relief of pain. A large boil may cause fever or flu-like symptoms, and often lymph glands in the area will enlarge as tender swellings under the skin. (see *Lumps in the skin*)

HOME TREATMENT
A boil may discharge and get better on its own. Keep it covered with a dressing if it is discharging; otherwise it will heal better if exposed to the air. **Magnesium sulphate paste** from the chemist is a messy old-fashioned but cheap remedy that is still popular. Whether it really helps is uncertain.

DOCTOR'S TREATMENT
In the very early stages, the first day or two when the boil is nothing more than a solid, slightly raised area of skin, a course of antibiotics may provide a speedy cure.

❖   ❖   ❖

Once pus has started to build up, antibiotics aren't likely to help, and the only treatment is by surgical drainage. Don't be tempted to try to lance a boil yourself – the chances are that you wouldn't be able to make a big enough hole to let out all the pus. A doctor would make a large cut, under local or general anaesthetic, and try to scrape out as much dead tissue and pus as possible from inside the boil. Choosing the right time to do this, when the boil is pointing, is crucial.

RECURRENT BOILS that keep appearing, often in crops all over your child's skin, can be a real problem. Boys seem more prone to them than girls, particularly as they reach adolescence. Occasionally other diseases, such as diabetes, eczema or blood disorders, are to blame, so SEE YOUR DOCTOR, who may suggest blood and urine tests to rule these out.

Usually there is no obvious cause and the problem seems to be that some people carry **staphylococcus**, the bacterium that causes boils, on their skin all the time. The carrier may be a different member of the family, who for some reason isn't prone to boils himself or herself. Or the child may carry the bacteria, continually reinfecting his or her skin and triggering boils.

DOCTOR'S TREATMENT
Treatment aims to get rid of these bugs. Quite often they lurk inside the nose, and your doctor may suggest treating everyone in the family with an antibiotic nasal cream. Your child may need a long course of antibiotics by mouth for around six weeks to clear the infection, and should have a bath every day using an antiseptic soap. Healthy diet and

exercise may also be advised. Recurrent boils are often a sign of being generally run down.

A CARBUNCLE is simply a group of boils close together which have merged into one large red, pus-filled area which will point, and discharge pus, from several different places. Carbuncles aren't easy to treat, even with surgery, and you should SEE YOUR DOCTOR.

❖   ❖   ❖   ❖   ❖

GUIDANCE
SEE YOUR DOCTOR if

❖   your child has recurrent boils or a carbuncle, OR

❖   he or she has had a nasty boil before, and is in the very early stages of another one, OR

❖   he or she has a boil that is painful and pointing, but which hasn't burst on its own.

Some GPs will drain boils themselves; most don't, and your best bet might be to go straight to the local casualty department.

BOW LEGS

Bow-legged toddlers are quite normal. Between the ages of one and three, most children's legs bow outwards at the knee; the opposite pattern develops over the next couple of years as knock-knees appear, eventually followed by the graceful legs of youth.

This bowing always disappears, and there is no need for any treatment.

TOES POINTING INWARDS is quite common in toddlers. Sometimes, besides being bowed, the tibia – the thick bone in the lower part of the leg – is twisted too. This has the effect of turning the child's feet so that the toes point inwards. It often leads to the familiar sight of toddlers tripping over their own feet because their toes overlap as they try to run. It is called **tibial torsion** and generally gets better by the age of three or four years.

Much more rarely, other problems are to blame for bow legs.

RICKETS softening of the bones due to a deficiency in Vitamin D, is rare nowadays, particularly as several foods such as flour and margarine have added Vitamin D. Asian children do seem more at risk.

DAMAGE TO THE BONE from injury or infection can cause permanent deformity. Often, this will affect just one leg, and although one leg is often quite normally a little more bowed than the other, you should SEE YOUR DOCTOR if the difference is marked. Occasionally, other rare bone diseases are to blame, too.

❖   ❖   ❖   ❖   ❖

GUIDANCE
SEE YOUR DOCTOR if

❖   your toddler's bow legs are still obvious after the age of three years, OR

- ✦ his or her toes point inwards very obviously. (There isn't likely to be any treatment, but the doctor will check for other conditions – such as a deformity of the bones of the foot – that may need surgery (see ***Foot problems***), OR

- ✦ one leg is very different from the other.

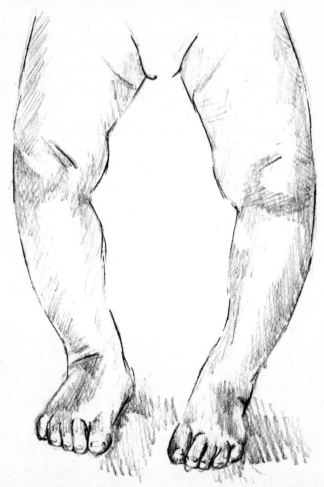

See your doctor if bow legs aren't better by the age of three, or if one leg is worse than the other

BREATH, BAD

Bad breath in children usually clears within a day or two; a longer-lasting problem is much more rare.

ILLNESS of any kind, usually an infection, is probably the most common cause. The child is obviously unwell, with a fever and the other symptoms of whichever illness is to blame. Many children seem to develop bad breath right at the start of an illness, and parents learn to recognise it as a sign that all is not well.

Sore throats and tonsillitis are particularly likely to cause foul breath as smelly pus forms on the tonsils at the back of the child's throat. More rarely an infection in the child's chest will give the same result. Coughs, colds and runny noses can all contribute too. Once the illness or infection is over, his or her breath should return to normal.

Food that the child eats can, of course, affect his or her breath in the same way as with adults, although less commonly as most children are not keen on spicy or highly flavoured foods. Again, the problem shouldn't last longer than a day or two.

BAD BREATH FOR A LONGER PERIOD may be the result of tooth decay, or more likely decaying fragments of food caught between the child's teeth. Gum infections may result, prolonging the problem by causing smelly pockets of pus to form between the teeth and gums.

HOME TREATMENT
It isn't always easy to clear all the fragments of food from the crowded teeth in a child's mouth, but it is important to do what you can. Antiseptic mouthwashes may help a little for older children, but regular brushing with a fluoride toothpaste is the most important treatment by far. If the problem continues then CHECK WITH YOUR DENTIST.

BAD BREATH WITH A RUNNY NOSE may point to something up a nostril that shouldn't be there. Small children are notorious for putting things up their noses and forgetting about them. After a day or two the nostril will start to discharge thick yellow mucus, and the child's breath may smell quite terrible (see *Foreign objects*).

Rhinitis, a runny nose due to allergy or simply because the child is prone to it, may be another cause. SEE YOUR DOCTOR: treatment such as steroid nasal sprays may be quite effective.

❖   ❖   ❖   ❖   ❖

GUIDANCE
Treatment depends on the cause; usually meticulous care about cleaning teeth, especially when the child is ill, is all you can do.

❖   ❖   ❖

SEE YOUR DOCTOR if there is a discharge from the nose, especially from just one side; or if your child is ill (see *Ill – should your child see the doctor?*).

BREATH-HOLDING

Around one or two per cent of toddlers are disposed to terrifying their parents by holding their breath, and refusing to take another.

These **breath-holding attacks** are in fact, completely harmless, and the child will always start breathing again. But they can be very frightening and at the time it may not be easy to convince yourself that they are harmless.

Usually, pain or frustration will set off an attack. Your toddler screams or cries, then holds his or her breath and becomes red in the face. Some will start breathing again at this stage; others may wait until their red face has turned quite blue, or even until they actually become unconscious.

LOSING CONSCIOUSNESS isn't too common during a breath-holding attack, but it may occur and it doesn't suggest that anything else is wrong. As soon as he or she passes out, your toddler will start breathing again and won't usually be out for more than a few seconds. If he or she is unconscious for longer, treat the child as if he or she had fainted (see *Fainting*).

TWITCHING OF THE ARMS AND LEGS can be an alarming symptom, too. Shortage of oxygen to the brain is the cause of passing out during an attack, and the same oxygen lack may cause brief twitching. Again, this is harmless and will stop, but if there is any doubt, you may need to CHECK WITH YOUR DOCTOR to be sure that epilepsy isn't to blame.

❖   ❖   ❖   ❖   ❖

GUIDANCE
Treatment doesn't really have much to offer; most doctors

think that it is best to do nothing. Some parents find that a sprinkling of cold water at the beginning of an attack will persuade a reluctant toddler to take a breath. Drugs from the doctor don't have anything to offer. Although breath-holding is most common around the ages of 18 months to two years, the attacks generally disappear soon after the age of three.

✧ ✧ ✧

SEE YOUR DOCTOR if

✤ Your toddler's attacks aren't exactly as described, OR

✤ He or she loses consciousness for more than a couple of seconds, OR

✤ Your toddler wets himself or herself or bites the tongue during an attack; or thrashes or jerks the arms or legs. These may be signs of epilepsy (see *Fits*).

A child whose attacks haven't disappeared by the age of three years, should probably be checked out by the doctor, too.

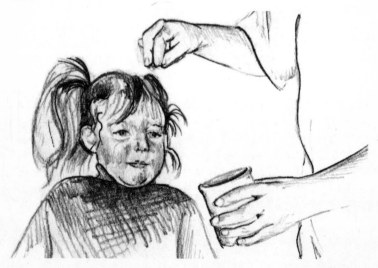

Sometimes a sprinkle of cold water will end a breath holding attack

BREATHING, NOISY OR DIFFICULT

DIFFICULT BREATHING, whatever the cause, should be CHECKED BY A DOCTOR IMMEDIATELY. The signs aren't always obvious; look for a faster breathing rate than usual, and whether your child is straining to breathe by tensing other muscles in the neck and chest as he or she breathes.

If the skin between or just under the ribs becomes sucked inwards as the child breathes in, there may be a **serious obstruction**. Another warning sign may be if the child is holding onto a table or chair, to brace the arms so that he or she can use muscles around the neck and shoulders to help take a breath. Turning blue is a serious sign of lack of oxygen which should be treated as an emergency.

These symptoms usually mean an obstruction to your child's breathing, or a problem with the lungs themselves such as infection.

NOISY BREATHING often means a partial blockage in the small air passages of the lungs or in the windpipe or throat. It needn't indicate a serious obstruction – ordinary coughs and colds, particularly in small babies, can cause horrendous noises without any danger.

RATTLY NOISES BREATHING IN AND OUT often come from the nose and throat of babies and children with colds. Babies are particularly prone to this, as the tiny passages in their nose and throat block with mucus so easily. Very young babies can't breathe through their mouths, except by crying, and so will make all kinds of noises as they struggle to breath through their noses. But provided that there are none of the signs of difficult breathing, and that your child isn't ill (see *Ill – should your child see the doctor?*), you can safely treat as you would a cold (see *Colds*).

NOISE WHEN BREATHING IN is called **inspiratory stridor**, and generally indicates a blockage in the throat or windpipe. This may be more serious, and should be CHECKED BY A DOCTOR. Sometimes an object which has gone down the wrong way and lodged in the child's windpipe is to blame.

Another possible cause is **epiglottitis**, an infection of the epiglottis at the back of the child's throat. The epiglottis is a flap of cartilage that normally closes the entrance to the windpipe during swallowing, to prevent food going down the wrong way.

A child with epiglottitis is likely to become suddenly hot and unwell with a sore throat and a croupy cough (see *Cough, hoarse or croupy*). He or she may be unable to swallow anything, including his or her own saliva, and so dribble constantly. Breathing will be noisy and the child may have the signs of difficult breathing above. Often, simple croup, rather than epiglottitis, is to blame, but don't take chances; epiglottitis can cause life-threatening blockage of the windpipe. SEE YOUR DOCTOR IMMEDIATELY.

A few babies have inspiratory stridor from birth, due to floppy cartilage in the wall of their larynx (voice box). This doesn't usually cause any problems, and disappears as the larynx develops properly.

NOISE WHEN BREATHING OUT is often wheeze – a high-pitched musical sound that comes from the tiny air passages of the lungs themselves rather than the windpipe or throat (see *Wheezing*).

❖　　　❖　　　❖　　　❖　　　❖

DOCTOR'S TREATMENT
SEE YOUR DOCTOR if your child has difficulty breathing, wheezing or stridor, or is ill (see *Ill – should your child see the doctor?*). Treatment will depend on the cause.

Wheezing may need treatment for infection or asthma (see *Wheezing*).

Stridor due to an inhaled object may respond to first aid measures (see *Foreign objects*).

Epiglottitis generally means hospital admission for antibiotics and, if necessary, a tube passed down the throat to relieve the obstruction.

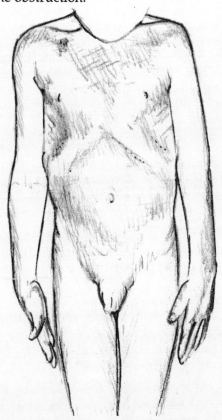

Sucking in of the skin under the ribs and bracing with the arms may be serious signs

35

BURNS AND SCALDS

Burns and scalds of children really should be taken quite seriously. As a general rule they may well be more serious than they seem.

About 12 per cent of accidental deaths in children under five, in this country, are caused by burns, and five per cent of deaths in older children. Burns and scalds are so dangerous because they can cause a loss of body fluid. Small children have a greater surface area of skin for their size compared to adults. Since fluid is lost through damaged skin, this gives scope for greater fluid loss – and of course children don't have as much body fluid in reserve in the first place.

Any burn or scald involving more than ten per cent of the child's skin will need hospital treatment, probably with a drip feeding fluid into a vein. This is equivalent to approximately the whole of an arm of most of a leg, or the whole of the head. As a rough guide, the area of your child's palm is about one per cent of his or her total skin area.

Even much smaller burns and scalds may still need hospital treatment to prevent the danger of scarring or infection.

SCALDS from hot liquid are more common than burns. They are usually the result of the child spilling a hot drink (or a parent spilling the drink with a child on his or her lap); pulling the flex of an electric kettle or the handle of a saucepan; or sitting in a very hot bath.

Fortunately scalds are usually less serious than burns, although they are likely to become more serious the longer the hot liquid stays in contact with the skin – so it is important to remove any clothing immediately.

BURNS are more likely to be caused by a child grabbing a hot object such as an electric fire, cooker ring or iron. Much larger burns are often the result of clothing catching fire.

GUIDANCE
How serious a burn or scald is can be very difficult to assess, particularly at first. The general rule is that all burns or scalds, except for the smallest, should be CHECKED BY A DOCTOR.

Most are **partial thickness burns**, meaning that only the surface skin layers are damaged. The deep skin layers aren't affected and the skin should eventually grow back normally without scarring.

❖   ❖   ❖

Blisters are common with partial thickness burns; the skin becomes red but pressing with a finger will produce a pale spot. The burn is likely to be painful because the nerves carrying pain sensation, deep in the skin, haven't been damaged.

FULL THICKNESS BURNS are more serious. The deeper layers of the skin have been damaged and when the burn does eventually heal it will leave a scar. Blisters are less common. **BLACK OR CHARRED SKIN,** or **LOSING THE SENSATION OF PAIN FROM THE BURNED AREA** are serious signs, but a full thickness burn isn't always easy to spot at first. All full thickness burns should be treated in hospital, and may need skin graft operations to heal properly.

HOME TREATMENT
This really means first aid, and deciding WHETHER TO SEE A DOCTOR. Get the child away from the source of the burn or scald and take off clothing that has been splashed with wet liquid, or that has caught fire. If, in a serious burn, the child's hair or clothing is on fire, then first wrap him or her in something like a blanket or coat to extinguish the fire.

❖   ❖   ❖

Cold water will soothe small partial thickness burns and scalds. Even small burns may be very painful, so a painkiller such as paracetamol is useful too (see dosage, page 11). If a burn doesn't need a doctor's attention it is usually best to leave it exposed to the air to heal – don't try to apply a dressing yourself.

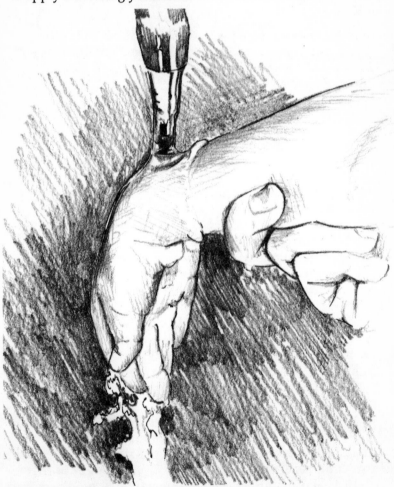

Holding a burn or scald under running cold water may provide immediate relief

❖   ❖   ❖   ❖   ❖

GUIDANCE

SEE YOUR DOCTOR for anything except the most minor burns and scalds. An area of redness bigger than a 2p piece, or any suspicion of a full thickness burn, should be checked. Don't be afraid to seek advice even for smaller burns – they could be more serious than they look, and it is best to make sure.

DOCTOR'S TREATMENT

This will probably involve puncturing any blisters and applying an antiseptic cream and sterile dressing, unless the burn is small in which case he may simply suggest leaving it exposed.

Large burns involving over ten per cent of the skin area, or full thickness burns, will mean a spell in hospital.

PREVENTION

Prevention is the most important aspect of dealing with burns. Use cooker and fire guards, turn saucepan handles inwards, and don't leave hot drinks or other liquids where young children could possibly reach them. Adjust the thermostat on your water heating system if water from the hot tap is at a scalding temperature. Radiators that are too hot can pose a danger too. Your health visitor should be able to provide you with more advice and leaflets.

CHOKING

Choking means that the windpipe has become blocked and the child can't breathe in, usually for a few moments.

SUDDEN CHOKING is most common and is often the result of an object in the child's mouth becoming lodged at the entrance to the windpipe (see *Foreign objects*).

SORE THROATS may make swallowing difficult, and the tonsils at the back of the child's throat may become hugely swollen, but will very rarely cause choking. A sore throat with epiglottitis (see *Breathing, noisy or difficult*) is a different matter and may cause severe breathing difficulty.

FOOD OR DRINK GOING DOWN THE WRONG WAY is a common cause of choking usually lasting only a few seconds. Don't be tempted to pat your child on the back as this may encourage food to fall into his or her windpipe. Usually coughing will clear the obstruction; if not then holding your child upside down may help, though often at the expense of losing everything he or she has just eaten (see *Foreign objects*).

CHOKING ON VOMIT or **CHOKING ON HIS OR HER OWN TONGUE** are fortunately rare in children, and although these terms are often used, they are actually rather misleading. The danger occurs only if the child is unconscious and lying on his or her back, when vomit or even the tongue may fall back to obstruct the throat. The danger is minimised by lying an unconscious child in the proper position on his or her side (see *Fainting*).

PROLONGED CHOKING over weeks or months since birth is more rare, but should be taken seriously. There are a

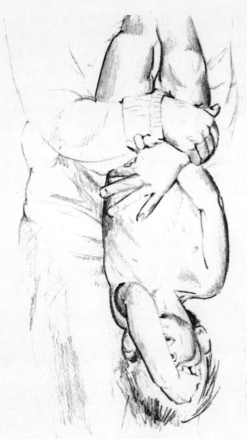

Holding a small child upside down may stop severe choking

large number of possible causes, including defects such as cleft palate or abnormal development of the tongue, throat, oesophagus (gullet) or jaw. Brain damage or cerebral palsy may affect the nerves and muscles that control swallowing, making it difficult. A few perfectly normal children don't seem to learn to control these muscles properly for several weeks or months.

SEVERE CHOKING IN A NEWBORN BABY may indicate serious disease such as an oesophagus (gullet) that hasn't developed properly, which will prevent normal feeding.

41

❖   ❖   ❖   ❖   ❖

GUIDANCE
SEE YOUR DOCTOR if your child has repeated bouts of choking or chokes from birth.

❖   ❖   ❖

Treatment for sudden choking depends on the cause (see *Foreign objects* and *Breathing, noisy or difficult*), but SEEK MEDICAL HELP STRAIGHT AWAY if your child has difficulty breathing for more than a few seconds.

CLUMSINESS

Around five to 15 school children in a hundred seem to be unusually clumsy. For some reason boys seem more often affected than girls. They are slow to learn to dress and can't manage buttons, zips or shoelaces. As toddlers, they aren't very good at feeding themselves and may make a terrible mess. They don't do well at tasks requiring fine coordination such as handwriting, drawing or jigsaws. They aren't good at games and PE and may fall or knock things over on a regular basis.

Some of the above list will seem familiar to any parent of perfectly normal children. When children are growing rapidly they can't always judge the position of their changing limbs, and mistakes are frequent. Growth spurts, particularly in adolescence, are often to blame. All this is quite normal, but really clumsy children seem to have problems all the time.

The cause of clumsiness like this really isn't known, although it may be that there are several possible causes. Everyone's skill with fine tasks is different, and many are probably simply quite normal children who aren't blessed with good coordination ability.

Other children may actually have a slight degree of **brain damage**. One possible cause is lack of oxygen to the baby during birth, although nowadays many doctors don't believe that this is as important as they used to think. Other factors, such as influences on the baby in the womb, may be more important. Certainly some clumsy children do seem to have learning and reading difficulties too, and a few have other signs of brain damage, such as a mild degree of cerebral palsy (weakness affecting part of the body due to brain damage).

HOME TREATMENT
Treatment really depends on just how severe the problem is.

Certainly all children respond to being encouraged to practise fine tasks at home, and vigorous encouragement can work wonders for many clumsy children. Often it pays to concentrate on areas where the child has difficulty.

DOCTOR'S TREATMENT
Children who are quite markedly clumsy should, ideally, be assessed by a doctor who may involve a team including teachers and physiotherapists. Again, treatment means exercises concentrating on areas of difficulty, but these are carefully worked out with regard to what the child is capable of.

Usually coordination improves quite well.

COLDS

The symptoms of a cold are familiar: a blocked and runny nose, streaming eyes, maybe a fever, headache and generally feeling unwell. Adults catch an average of four colds a year, although children have more than their share as they haven't developed immunity to the viruses responsible. School children can expect six to eight colds each year.

COLDS IN BABIES may appear quite alarming as the air passages in a baby's nose are tiny, and easily become blocked. Young babies don't know how to breathe through their mouths except by crying, so a blocked nose produces either crying or the most astonishing snuffling and snorting as the child tries to breathe. Older babies may have trouble feeding as they can't breathe through the blocked nose and suck with the mouth at the same time.

Alarming as this can appear, it doesn't indicate a serious problem. The worst that is likely to happen, if the baby's nose completely blocks, is that he or she will wake up (if asleep) and start to cry.

TODDLERS know how to breathe through their mouths, and have bigger noses, so blockage isn't usually a problem. Phlegm in their throats may rattle and is often mistaken for a chest infection, although usually, if you listen carefully, you can be sure that the noise is all coming from the throat.

OLDER CHILDREN generally have similar symptoms to those of adults.

❖   ❖   ❖   ❖   ❖

GUIDANCE
The cause of colds is a virus infection. There are over 100 different cold viruses, and once you have been infected by one, you develop immunity and will never be infected by it again. Unfortunately, cold viruses are constantly changing,

so there is nothing to stop you encountering the same virus in a different form the next year and becoming reinfected.

❖   ❖   ❖

Treatment means controlling the symptoms. There is no generally available treatment against the viruses that cause colds, or which will make colds better any more quickly. Antibiotic drugs are only effective against infections caused by bacteria; although they have no effect against the viruses that cause colds, they may occasionally be needed if your child develops complications from a cold, in which case, SEE YOUR DOCTOR.

❖   ❖   ❖

Controlling the symptoms means using paracetamol to control pain or fever in children and babies over two months of age (see dosage, page 11). **Decongestant nose drops** such as xylometazoline, available from your chemist, can help to clear a blocked nose, although they aren't recommended for babies under three months. SEE YOUR DOCTOR, who may suggest sterile saline nose drops for younger ages.

❖   ❖   ❖

For nose drops to work, it is important to use them properly. Place your child face up on your lap with the feet towards you and the head hanging over your knees. An older child can lie on the bed with his or her head hanging over the edge.

Put one or two drops in each nostril, and keep the child's head down for a couple of minutes while they soak in. This may produce a noisy protest, but will give the drops a chance to work.

❖   ❖   ❖

Steam helps too, by aiding the drainage of mucus and phlegm and easing the pain of a sore dry nose and throat.

Try letting a (closely supervised) electric kettle boil in the bedroom for a few minutes before bedtime or, if you have radiators, put wet towels over them to produce some steam overnight. Letting the child play by day in steamy places such as in a bathroom or kitchen, may help.

❖   ❖   ❖

Aromatic rubs or capsules may help, particularly if mixed with steam, but they don't usually offer much extra benefit. Other cold cures, generally, don't seem to have much advantage over these simple remedies.

❖   ❖   ❖

Food may not interest a child suffering from a cold. This doesn't matter, although it is important to keep the child drinking; hot drinks and fruit juices seem to go down best.

Bottle-fed babies who go off their milk can happily stick to water or juice for a few days.

❖   ❖   ❖

The duration of a cold is usually around five days to a week. The child is most infectious to others for the first couple of days. Snuffly noses may take a long time to return completely to normal, especially in small babies who may remain snuffly for a couple of weeks or more.

❖   ❖   ❖

SEE YOUR DOCTOR if there is a possibility that the cold may have developed a complication, such as a chest or ear infection. This may mean that your child

❖   becomes ill (see *Ill – should your child see the doctor?*), OR

❖   develops earache (possibility of an ear infection – see *Pain or discharge in the ear*), OR

❖   vomits or won't drink anything at all (could be general signs of a secondary infection anywhere), OR

47

- ❖ has rapid breathing (possibility of a chest infection), OR

- ❖ becomes unwell with a fever, several days after the cold has started (could be any secondary infection), OR

- ❖ makes wheezing noises when breathing out (possibility of asthma or chest infection – see *Wheezing*), OR

- ❖ makes hoarse noises or has difficulty in breathing (could be epiglottitis – see *Breathing, noisy or difficult*).

In general, however, a cold in a child is no more serious than a cold in an adult, and will end after a few days of misery.

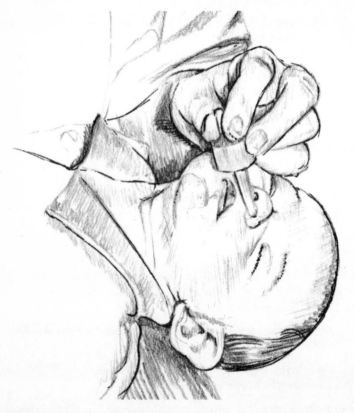

Keep your child's head down for a minute or two as the drops soak in

COLIC

Colic covers a multitude of sins. Parents know just what they mean when they describe an attack of colic in their baby, but nobody knows what is really going on. In fact, there may be different problems in different babies, all lumped together under the same term, colic.

THREE MONTH COLIC or **EVENING COLIC** are terms used to describe a general pattern.

Babies vary enormously in their amount of crying, but most cry more and more during the day until the age of around three months, when their crying reaches a peak (see *Crying babies*). Afterwards, most babies start to cry less. Sometimes the crying occurs mainly in the evening.

❖   ❖   ❖

Colic means pain from spasm of part of the bowel, and often it does seem as if that is what is going on. Your baby may suddenly screw up his or her face and cry, maybe lifting the legs or producing a dirty nappy or wind from either end – which sometimes seems to bring some relief.

However, the truth is that nobody really knows what does cause the pain – or even whether the baby is in pain at all, although it does often look like it. It is likely that there is more than one cause. Some babies' crying doesn't seem to be related to bowel problems, for example, but settles if they are changed or cuddled or fed.

❖   ❖   ❖

Often there may be more than one problem going on at once. Sometimes stress can make matters worse. A crying baby can be a tremendous physical and emotional strain, and not surprisingly causes upset and anxiety. Unfortunately, babies are remarkably good at picking up even slight signs of tension from their parents. They react by crying even more, and may not feed well. This sets up a vicious circle of tension and crying that it can be hard to break.

This isn't the same as saying that colic is an emotional or psychological problem, but emotion can sometimes contribute to the overall picture.

GUIDANCE
Treatment of colic has to take account of the different problems that may be going on. Usually this means experimentation, trying a variety of remedies until you find one that suits you and your baby. Because nobody really knows what is at the root of the problem, this is the only way to find out.

❖   ❖   ❖

Your health visitor will be experienced in dealing with colic and crying, and should be able to offer help and suggestions.

❖   ❖   ❖

Try the effect of picking your baby up when he or she cries, putting him or her down, feeding, changing, winding, carrying around, keeping him or her still, going for a walk, going for a drive. Try anything that might help.

❖   ❖   ❖

Colic drops such as Infacol, available from your chemist, sometimes help by reducing the amount of gas in your baby's stomach.

Avoiding cow's milk seems to produce a dramatic improvement in some babies. This may mean changing to a soya bean based formula if you are bottle feeding, or avoiding dairy products yourself if you are breast-feeding. Ask your health visitor for advice before making this kind of change to your diet.

Again, it seems difficult to predict which babies will respond to which treatments without simply giving them a try.

❖ ❖ ❖

Whatever it really is, colic doesn't last for ever and usually improves rapidly after around three months. And it isn't a sign of harm or damage to your baby.

❖ ❖ ❖

SEE YOUR DOCTOR if your baby's crying suddenly increases or becomes different from usual. In this way you can ensure that there isn't another cause (see *Crying babies*), which should not be blamed on colic.

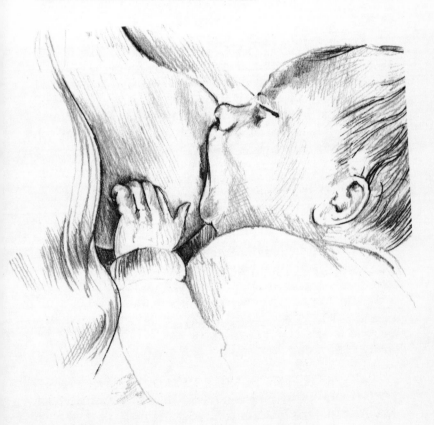

Avoiding dairy products sometimes helps colic

CONSTIPATION

Constipation is really a description of what happens when your child visits the loo rather than how many times he or she uses it. It is quite normal to open the bowels anything from once every three days to three times a day, and simply not going very often doesn't necessarily mean constipation.

Straining on the loo, eventually to produce a small amount of hard stool, is much more significant. Although bouts of constipation like this are common in children, they can cause lasting problems if they are prolonged.

A BOUT OF CONSTIPATION FOR A SHORT TIME isn't likely to suggest anything serious. It may follow any illness where your child's appetite hasn't been up to scratch, particularly an episode of diarrhoea or vomiting where fluid has been lost from the bowel. It may be due to a sudden change in diet, and is common in small babies especially if they are breast-fed or aren't taking enough fluid.

Generally the problem will right itself in a short time. Rarely, a more serious problem such as intestinal blockage is to blame.

GUIDANCE
Treatment isn't usually necessary for a brief bout of constipation, although you should SEE YOUR DOCTOR if your child has pain around his or her anus (possibility of an anal fissure) or has tummy pain or is vomiting (possibility of intestinal blockage). Constipation in babies will usually respond to lots of pure fruit juice, and in older children to plenty of fibre and fluid.

CONSTIPATION BECAUSE A CHILD DOESN'T WANT TO LET GO is also quite common. Children starting school may find that the loos are cold, aren't private, or they may not quite be able to manage on their own. Some may become convinced there are monsters in the loo at home.

Sometimes, an embarrassing accident in the pants will lead the child to try to hold his or her stool in to avoid a recurrence. Sometimes a temporary bout of constipation will cause an **anal fissure** – a tear in the skin around the anus (see *Blood in the stools*) which will make opening the bowels very painful.

For any of these reasons the child tries to hold the stool in, rather than opening the bowels when he or she needs to. Faeces build up in the rectum and become hard, making the child even more anxious to try to avoid the fateful moment when the bowels must be opened.

CONSTIPATION FOR A LONG PERIOD OF TIME often starts in the above way. **Diet** may be another cause, particularly if there isn't much roughage (fruit, veg and fibre) and the child is filling up with milk.

DISEASES OF THE BOWEL are occasionally to blame. For example, Hirschprung's disease is a condition where the nerve supply to the child's rectum hasn't developed properly, and anorectal stenosis is a narrowing of the child's anus. Both these conditions are present from birth and usually cause quite severe constipation from a very early age. Occasionally, there are other causes, such as cerebral palsy (brain damage at birth).

LOSS OF CONTROL OVER BOWEL MOVEMENTS may follow long-term constipation. As hard faeces build up, the child's rectum – the part of the bowel which stores the stool just before it reaches his anus – becomes stretched. The stretched muscles in the wall of the rectum can't work properly, and the child may start to lose control over the bowel and have accidents.

Another problem is that liquid faeces may start to leak around the hard stool in the rectum and out through the child's anus. It may even look as if it is diarrhoea, that the child can't control, although the cause is really constipation.

❖　　　❖　　　❖　　　❖　　　❖

GUIDANCE
Treatment of long-term constipation, lasting more than a few weeks, may be more involved than that for a brief bout. As a general rule you should always SEE YOUR DOCTOR first. The doctor will examine your child's abdomen for sings of accumulated faeces, and may need to examine your child's rectum with a finger too. This is quite safe, even in the tiniest babies, and although a little uncomfortable shouldn't hurt (unless your child has an anal fissure, which the doctor may be able to spot simply by looking).

DOCTOR'S TREATMENT
This will depend on what the doctor finds on examining your child. The possibility of Hirschprung's disease or anorectal stenosis would lead to a hospital referral and possibly surgery. Constipation due to holding on, or an anal fissure, may get better after a course of laxative drugs. Occasionally hospital referral, and surgery to stretch the anus is necessary.

❖   ❖   ❖

Often a star chart similar to those used in bed wetting (see *Bed wetting*) will reward the child for using the loo properly and help to retrain him or her to use the bowel muscles properly.

❖   ❖   ❖

A combination of treatments may be required, but almost always the problem can be helped ultimately.

COUGH AND COLD

Colds often bring coughs as well as all the other symptoms of misery to children (see *Colds*). Usually this is no more than what is expected; occasionally there are other symptoms which may suggest that there is something else going on.

THE COUGHING is due to phlegm that drips down the back of the nose to the throat. This irritates the top of the child's windpipe and triggers his or her **cough reflex** – designed to prevent anything finding its way down the windpipe into the lungs.

The phlegm is coughed up into the child's mouth, and it may look as if he or she is coughing up large amounts from the lungs. Phlegm in the throat may rattle as the child breathes, giving the impression of chestiness too, but the problem is all in the nose and throat, and the symptoms don't suggest any problem in the chest.

The cough may be prolonged, lasting a week or two after the cold itself has got better. Smokers in the household may cause an even more prolonged cough.

GUIDANCE
Treatment for this cough is really similar to general treatment for a cold (see *Colds*). Cough mixtures from the chemist may sometimes be useful particularly at night-time, but often aren't tremendously effective. Although they may help to suppress the symptoms, they won't actually clear up the cough any more quickly. A **steamy atmosphere** often helps (see *Colds*).

❖   ❖   ❖

SEE YOUR DOCTOR if you think that your child's cough may suggest something more than just a cold. Check whether your child is ill (see *Ill – should your child see the doctor?*), or has rapid breathing. This may suggest **a chest infection** – particularly if he or she becomes more ill and feverish several days after the cold first started.

CHEST INFECTIONS are actually uncommon with straightforward coughs and colds. An infection may be **lobar pneumonia**, affecting only one part of the lung, or **bronchitis** or **bronchopneumonia**, which affect most of both lungs.

PNEUMONIA, or **LOBAR PNEUMONIA**, usually affects schoolchildren around the ages of four to ten years. The child may become quite suddenly ill with a fever, often vomiting, and a pain on one side of the chest. (Sometimes the pain seems to be in the upper part of the abdomen, instead.) He or she will seem quite unwell and will breathe fast, sometimes with a grunt at the end of each breath out. Usually, there is a cough, but sometimes there may be none at all. Coughing or breathing will tend to make the pain worse (see **pleuritic pain** in *Pain in the chest*).

SEE YOUR DOCTOR if you suspect pneumonia. Treatment with antibiotics usually produces a dramatic improvement.

BRONCHITIS is actually rather a vague term when referring to children. It means an infection all over the lungs, but doctors now realise that many children who used to be diagnosed with bronchitis were really suffering from **asthma** (see *Wheezing*), and not from an infection at all.

BRONCHOPNEUMONIA usually affects babies and toddlers, sometimes after a bout of measles or whooping cough. The child develops a dry cough and rapid breathing; over a day or two he or she may become quite ill (see *Ill – should your child see the doctor?*).

You should SEE YOUR DOCTOR if you suspect bronchopneumonia. Treatment is with antibiotic drugs, in hospital if necessary.

56

NOISES COMING FROM THE CHEST should be
CHECKED BY YOUR DOCTOR too, although often these
turn out to be coming from the child's throat once the doctor
listens through a stethoscope.

WHEEZING (see *Wheezing*) may indicate asthma or a chest
infection and should be CHECKED BY YOUR DOCTOR.

❖   ❖   ❖   ❖   ❖

Also SEE YOUR DOCTOR if the cough lasts for more than
two weeks, or if it occurs in one of the particular patterns
that may suggest that something else is going on. For
example, at night (see *Cough, night-time*), as a croupy cough
(see *Cough, hoarse or croupy*), or in spasms (see *Cough, in
spasms or whooping*).

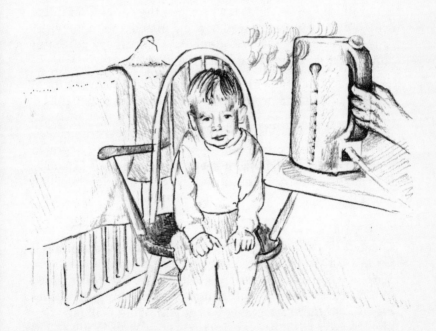

A steamy atmosphere may help to relieve cough and cold symptoms

COUGH, HOARSE OR CROUPY

The cough of croup, once heard, is never forgotten. It is a hoarse, barking, dry cough which sounds a little like a performing seal.

CROUP is caused by a virus infection of the child's throat, larynx (voice box) and windpipe. Swelling and irritation of the entrance to the windpipe causes the cough, and may lead to harsh rasping noises from the throat as the child breathes in.

Symptoms usually start quite suddenly with a fever and a generally miserable child, as well as the cough and noisy breathing. Adults may well become infected with the virus at the same time, but will develop an ordinary cold, not croup, as their larynx is so much bigger.

The duration of the child's illness isn't usually very long, generally not much more than a couple of days and nights.

A CROUPY COUGH doesn't always mean croup. Some children have a particular type of larynx and seem to develop croupy coughs whenever they have colds. Usually the cough will be quite mild, and the child shouldn't be ill in any other way.

GUIDANCE

Dangers of croup are generally small, although sometimes it isn't easy to tell the difference between croup and the more serious condition of **acute epiglottitis** (see *Breathing, noisy or difficult*). If any of the signs of breathing difficulty mentioned there are present, or if your child is ill (see *Ill – should your child see the doctor?*) you should SEE YOUR DOCTOR or take your child to casualty immediately.

❖   ❖   ❖

In fact, it is a good idea to SEE YOUR DOCTOR with any case of croup. This is particularly important if your child is aged less than one, or over four years. Although croup is most common between these ages, it can be more severe in younger or older children. The danger is the risk of blockage to the windpipe (see *Breathing, noisy or difficult*).

HOME TREATMENT
Treatment generally means steam. Encourage your child to play in a steamy kitchen or bathroom, and boil an electric kettle (closely supervised) in his or her room at night. If you have central heating, put wet towels over the radiators to make more steam. This helps to reduce the swelling and pain around your child's larynx, and seems to make breathing a little easier. Paracetamol (see dosage, page 11) is useful for pain and fever.

DOCTOR'S TREATMENT
Your doctor may prescribe antibiotics; although croup is a virus infection that won't respond to antibiotics, the doctor may want to guard against the possibility of epiglottitis.

❖   ❖   ❖

If your doctor has any doubt about the possibility of a breathing obstruction admission to hospital, for steam treatment and observation, may be suggested.

COUGH, IN SPASMS OR WHOOPING

Spasms of coughing are familiar to most people; entering a dusty, dry or smoky atmosphere may trigger them. Ordinary coughs due to a cold may occur in bouts, maybe triggered by something in the atmosphere. Sometimes the act of coughing itself causes inflammation and irritation of the throat and windpipe, setting off even more coughing – a vicious circle which may cause a coughing spasm for several minutes.

All this is quite normal, and shouldn't require any treatment other than ordinary treatment for coughs and colds. (see *Cough and cold*.) But sometimes spasms of coughing in a child are a sign of whooping cough.

WHOOPING COUGH can occur even in children who have had their jabs to protect against it. This is because there are two or three different bugs that can cause very similar symptoms. Although the jab usually gives very good protection against bordetella pertussis, the bacterium responsible for true whooping cough, it doesn't protect against the others.

This doesn't matter from the point of view of protecting your child – it is true whooping cough that is potentially dangerous, and against which your child should be **immunised**. But similar, although milder, infections are possible from the other bugs.

A COUGH IN SPASMS OFTEN FOLLOWED BY RETCHING OR VOMITING may mean whooping cough. The characteristic 'whoop' that the child makes as he or she takes the first breath after a cough, may confirm the diagnosis, although very young children often don't have this.

The spasms may be very powerful, the child coughing and coughing until there seems to be no breath left in his or her lungs and turning blue in the face before finally taking a breath with a loud whoop. Usually the cough is worse at night-time.

A COLD WITH RUNNY NOSE AND SLIGHT FEVER is often the first sign of whooping cough, before the cough develops a couple of days later.

A MILDER COUGH THAT LASTS FOR WEEKS OR MONTHS can follow whooping cough, and is one of the possible causes of a long-term cough (see *Cough, long-term*).

❖   ❖   ❖   ❖   ❖

GUIDANCE
SEE YOUR DOCTOR if you suspect whooping cough. Although there is no specific treatment, the doctor will check how serious the infection is, and may suggest a course of antibiotics to reduce the risk of infection to other children.

❖   ❖   ❖

Paracetamol is useful for pain or fever (see dosage, page 11); cough mixtures may help a little, and promethazine syrup from the chemist is a safe sedative which may be useful to control the cough at night.

COUGH, LONG-TERM

COUGHS LASTING LONGER THAN TWO OR THREE WEEKS may be perfectly harmless, but should generally be CHECKED BY A DOCTOR.

LONG-TERM COUGHING, MAINLY AT NIGHT raises the possibility of a tendency to asthma (see *Cough, night-time* and *Wheezing*).

❖   ❖   ❖

COUGHING SINCE BIRTH or a very early age, is unusual and may indicate a problem with the development of the baby's windpipe or even heart disease.

BABIES WHO COUGH WHEN FEEDING may have a problem with the valve between their gullet and stomach, causing them to regurgitate food which irritates their throat when they feed.

GUIDANCE
Any of these problems require expert assessment and treatment, possibly by surgery, so SEE YOUR DOCTOR.

COUGHS IN OLDER CHILDREN may not be very significant; the most likely explanation is often a prolonged cough following a cold, particularly if one or both parents smoke.

Many children go through what doctors describe as a **catarrhal phase** in their first few years of life; they catch one cold after another and have a cough and constantly blocked or runny nose between attacks. This is quite normal, as they are gradually developing immunity to the cold viruses they encounter. After a few years, their tendency to perpetual coughs and colds eventually gets better.

Other possibilities include **asthma** (see *Wheezing* and *Cough, night-time*) or a small object which has been breathed into one of the small air passages inside the child's lung (see *Foreign objects*).

A **chest or sinus infection** is another possibility, as is the aftermath of whooping cough (see *Cough, in spasms or whooping*). Some children develop a habit of coughing or clearing their throats, particularly when they are nervous, although there is nothing physically wrong.

Rarely, the child has a condition such as **cystic fibrosis**, which makes him or her prone to repeated chest infections and constant coughs.

❖   ❖   ❖   ❖   ❖

GUIDANCE
SEE YOUR DOCTOR if a cough has persisted for more than two or three weeks and especially if your child seems at all unwell, loses his or her appetite, loses weight or develops sweats and fevers (possibility of chest infections, including tuberculosis).

DOCTOR'S TREATMENT
Your doctor will examine your child's chest and may suggest a chest X-ray if necessary to rule out a problem such as infection or a foreign object.

❖   ❖   ❖

Treatment will depend on the cause but, if there doesn't seem to be very much wrong, it is likely to consist of nothing more than reassurance, advice to stop smoking if you do, and general advice for helping coughs (see *Cough and cold*).

COUGH, NIGHT-TIME

Most coughs seem to be worse at night. There are probably several reasons for this. One is that lying down flat doesn't allow mucus and phlegm in the nose and sinuses to drain as it should. Instead it builds up in the throat and triggers the cough reflex. Mucus and fluid in the lungs don't drain efficiently either, due to changes in the blood supply to the lungs while lying flat.

A cough when lying down is likely to be weaker than a cough when standing up, and is not as effective at clearing the throat of phlegm, so there is the need to cough more to achieve the same effect. And the air itself becomes colder and drier at night, causing more irritation to the throat and windpipe.

A COUGH WHICH IS MUCH WORSE AT NIGHT, OR ONLY OCCURS AT NIGHT may, however, mean that something else is going on. Asthma and whooping cough are strong possibilities; the aftermath of whooping cough may leave a persistent cough for weeks or even months (see *Cough, in spasms or whooping*).

ASTHMA in adults usually gives a characteristic wheeze when breathing out, together with a tight chest and difficulty in breathing (see *Wheezing*). The symptoms may be the same in children, but a night-time cough is common too. In children who are relatively mildly affected, it may be the only symptom. It is important to be sure whether asthma is the cause so SEE YOUR DOCTOR.

Besides the cough, a child who is affected in this way is likely to have other symptoms, even though they may not be obvious. He or she may cough or become quickly puffed when playing games, and may avoid them as a result. In fact, some children limit their range of day-to-day activity quite severely in this way without realising what they are doing. Asthma that isn't treated may affect growth, too (see *Wheezing*).

❖   ❖   ❖   ❖   ❖

GUIDANCE
Treatment of a night-time cough depends on the cause. Whooping cough will clear eventually (see *Cough, in spasms or whooping*); whereas treatment for asthma is generally very effective nowadays (see *Wheezing*).

❖   ❖   ❖

SEE YOUR DOCTOR if your child has a persistent cough that is worse at night or only occurs at night, as asthma is an important condition to diagnose. Occasionally the doctor may suggest a chest X-ray to rule out other problems (see *Cough, long-term*).

CRADLE CAP AND DANDRUFF

THE LIGHT BROWN CRUST OF DRY, DEAD SKIN over the baby's scalp, known as **cradle cap**, can look a bit of a mess but is common and quite harmless. In fact, cradle cap is part of the more widespread condition of **seborrhoeic dermatitis**.

Don't be confused by the words dermatitis and eczema; they both mean exactly the same thing. They mean dry, inflamed skin. So seborrhoeic eczema and seborrhoeic dermatitis are identical conditions. Seborrhoeic dermatitis is particularly common in babies, but older children and adults can be affected too.

Symptoms include cradle cap or, in order children, scurf and dandruff which may be quite severe. There may be a red, dry, slightly scaly rash on the child's forehead and cheeks and behind her or her ears. Sometimes the trunk, and occasionally arms and legs, are affected too.

GUIDANCE
The cause of seborrhoeic dermatitis and cradle cap isn't fully understood. Some babies just seem prone to it, particularly if they have inherited a tendency to sensitive skin. Babies whose parents suffer from eczema may be at greater risk, and although cradle cap and seborrhoeic dermatitis usually clear with a year or so, a few children may go on to develop childhood eczema (see *Rashes, long-term*).

❖   ❖   ❖

Fungus infections of the skin have recently been found to be an important cause of seborrhoeic dermatitis in adults. They are probably much less important in babies, although older children may sometimes respond well to anti-fungal therapy.

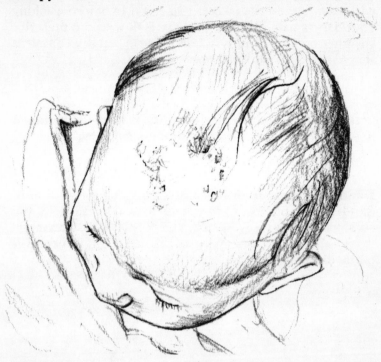

Cradle cap is part of the more widespread condition of seborrhoeic dermatitis

HOME TREATMENT

Treatment for **cradle cap** is usually straightforward. **Cradle cap shampoo** from your chemist will help to remove the dead scaly skin, and using it regularly may well be enough to keep your baby's scalp clear.

Rubbing the scalp with **olive oil** is a popular remedy, although this really only softens the dead skin making it easier to remove. Gentle rubbing with a damp flannel will often help to clear dead skin flakes.

❖   ❖   ❖

If special shampoos aren't enough then something stronger, such as **salicylic acid and sulphur cream** from your chemist will probably do the trick if you rub it in before washing your baby's hair. SEE YOUR DOCTOR who can prescribe stronger creams if all else fails. These usually contain a steroid such as hydrocortisone.

❖ ❖ ❖

Treatment for **seborrhoeic dermatitis** is likely to be similar to the treatment of eczema (see *Rashes, long-term*).

❖ ❖ ❖

Dandruff in older children often gets better with anti-dandruff shampoo or creams such as salicylic acid and sulphur, but if it is severe, SEE YOUR DOCTOR, who might try an anti-fungal shampoo in case a fungal infection is partly to blame.

CRYING BABIES

Babies vary enormously in the amount they cry. This variation is quite normal and most of the time it doesn't seem to have anything to do with your style of parenting.

Although there is such variation, as a general rule the amount of crying steadily increases over the first few weeks of a baby's life until it reaches a peak at around three months of age, after which it starts to decline. Sometimes the cause of the crying – hunger, pain or a dirty nappy – will be obvious. Often it isn't, and although the crying may be given a label such as colic, no one is really sure what is going on (see *Colic*).

BABIES WHO CRY ALL THE TIME can be an enormous strain both physically and emotionally. Guilt at not seeming able to care for your baby adequately, together with the nagging fear that there might be some serious or painful condition at the root of it all, can be intolerable.

GUIDANCE
These fears are groundless, but no less real for that. SEE YOUR DOCTOR, who should be able to reassure you that there is nothing physically wrong, and with time you should be able to work out various ways of helping the crying (see *Colic*).

❖   ❖   ❖

Don't be afraid to ask for help, and a good relationship with your health visitor can be invaluable – she is trained and experienced in helping you cope with just this kind of problem.

❖   ❖   ❖

Cry-sis is an organisation which offers a telephone support line, as well as a newsletter and advice on helpful books, to parents of crying or sleepless babies. You can contact them on 071-404 5011.

SUDDEN OR UNUSUAL CRYING IN BABIES who don't usually cry, is a different matter altogether. It is a common complaint, and often the cause is obvious.

GUIDANCE
If the cause is not obvious, look for **common causes of sudden crying**. These include hunger or thirst, a wet or dirty nappy, nappy rash, teething (suggested by dribbling and excessive chewing), and possibly even being too hot or cold.

❖   ❖   ❖

Check for a lump in the groin – hernias are quite common in babies – (see *Lumps, groin or testicle*) or swelling of the testicles in a boy – could mean a hernia, or a twisted testicle.

CRYING WHEN PASSING URINE seems to be quite normal in some babies but it should always be CHECKED BY A DOCTOR to rule out the possibility of a **urine infection**. Constipation in babies usually only causes pain and crying when they are actually passing a motion (see *Constipation*).

A LIKELY CAUSE OF SUDDEN CRYING is simply that your baby is coming down with an infection. This is more likely if he or she has a temperature or symptoms of a cough or cold, or enlarged glands in the neck or groin.

❖   ❖   ❖   ❖   ❖

GUIDANCE
Although minor infections will make babies and children miserable, they don't normally cause incessant, constant crying.

❖   ❖   ❖

If you can't find any of the causes mentioned above, then try to console your baby any way you can (see *Colic*). If your baby is still crying after an hour, then SEE YOUR DOCTOR IMMEDIATELY.

❖   ❖   ❖

If the cry doesn't sound like your baby's normal cry, if your baby is ill (see *Ill – should your child see the doctor?*), or there are other symptoms – such as vomiting or bloody bowel motions – then SEE YOUR DOCTOR WITHOUT DELAY.

DOCTOR'S TREATMENT
The doctor will check for the causes mentioned above and will also look for other common causes such as an ear infection (see *Pain or discharge in the ear*) or intussusception (a blockage of the bowel – suspect if your baby seems to have stomach pain, possibly drawing the legs up, with vomiting and bloody stools).

If the baby is in obvious distress and the doctor can't find a cause he or she may even suggest observation in hospital.

❖   ❖   ❖   ❖   ❖

As with colic, sudden crying is common in babies and very often there simply isn't an obvious cause. The crying usually vanishes as mysteriously as it appeared.

CUTS, SCRAPES AND BRUISES

Cuts and bruises are a normal part of a healthy, inquisitive childhood.

BRUISES THAT APPEAR FOR NO REASON are almost always the result of a bump or knock that has been forgotten.

If large numbers suddenly start to appear, or bruises crop up in areas such as the chest or abdomen that aren't usually prone to bumps, then CHECK WITH YOUR DOCTOR to rule out the rare possibility of a blood disorder.

ORDINARY BRUISES don't usually need any treatment.

A towel or flannel soaked in cold water may help to reduce the pain and swelling if you apply it in the first few hours of a bruise; it isn't likely to help much after this. Some people swear by **arnica**, a homeopathic remedy which you can buy from the chemist to apply to a bruise. Paracetamol will help reduce pain if necessary (see dosage, page 11).

BRUISING AROUND A JOINT may possibly be a sign of a broken bone (particularly elbow, wrist, shoulder, collar bone) or a joint sprain (ankle, wrist), even if the joint doesn't seem deformed or out of place. The heavier the blow or impact that caused the bruise, the more likely this is; children's bones should be perfectly resilient to the knocks and bumps of everyday life.

If your child can move the affected limb normally without pain then there probably isn't a problem; if not, or if the bruising is severe, then best to CHECK WITH YOUR DOCTOR.

A LARGE BRUISE WITH BROKEN SKIN should be watched for signs of infection – increasing swelling with

72

redness spreading from the centre. This is rare in children, but should be CHECKED BY YOUR DOCTOR if it occurs.

SCRAPES AND GRAZES don't usually need much treatment other than washing with soap and water. An antiseptic lotion may help. Cover the graze only if it is necessary to stop the bleeding or keep it clean; usually healing is quickest if it is exposed to the air.

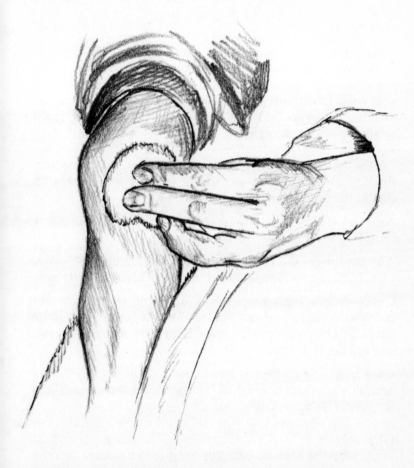

Bruising around a joint may be a sign of a broken bone

GUIDANCE
Don't worry about one or two specs of dirt that won't come out; they will work their way out as the skin heals. But if there are large amounts of deeply embedded dirt that you can't get out (sometimes a problem with tarmac from the road) you should TAKE YOUR CHILD TO CASUALTY; the doctors there may need to clean the area, possibly even under anaesthetic.

❖   ❖   ❖

Infection is more common with grazes and usually shows as spreading redness of the skin around the area, with sticky pus leaking from the graze itself. Regular cleaning with an antiseptic lotion will usually control the problem, but if the infection is severe, SEE YOUR DOCTOR, who may suggest treatment with antibiotics.

CUTS IN CHILDREN are usually shallow, and generally heal quickly. But any cut that is deeper than a scratch carries the risk of scarring when it heals.

Any cut on a child's face should be CHECKED BY A DOCTOR.

Any cut longer than two centimetres should be SEEN BY A DOCTOR, in case it would heal more quickly with stitches.

Cuts over **moving areas**, such as joints and tendons, or any cut whose edges you can't bring easily together, should be CHECKED BY A DOCTOR, even if the cuts are less than two centimetres in length.

Cuts from dog bites may need special treatment including antibiotics if there is a risk of infection, and should be SEEN BY A DOCTOR.

GUIDANCE
First, **stop the bleeding** by applying firm pressure directly on to the cut through a bandage or cloth. If necessary, keep this up for as long as 15 minutes – it will stop virtually any bleeding, including bleeding from arteries in severe

lacerations within this time. If the cut is still bleeding after 15 minutes, SEE A DOCTOR.

❖   ❖   ❖

If you do treat the cut yourself, first wash it with soap and water and make sure that the edges are clean, not ragged, and come together easily. An adhesive plaster will help small cuts; you can hold slightly larger ones together with sterile sticky strips of tape from your chemist. Keep the cut clean and dry while it heals, protecting it with a clean dressing if necessary.

❖   ❖   ❖

If you can't get the cut clean, the bleeding won't stop after 15 minutes, the edges are ragged or you can't keep the edges together, SEE A DOCTOR.

Usually this means going straight to casualty for cleaning and stitching or sticky strips, although some GPs will stitch cuts themselves.

❖   ❖   ❖

Infections are possible with any cut and if spreading redness and tenderness develops, then SEE YOUR DOCTOR.

Tetanus is an infection usually of deep cuts, which can lead to paralysis and death. It is rare in this country because the routine jabs given to all children protect against it. But it is important to keep your child up to date with his or her tetanus protection, with a booster jab every 10 years, for life.

DIARRHOEA

Doctors define diarrhoea as excessively runny stools, no matter how many times the child goes to the loo during the day. In fact, how often your child goes isn't very important – there is a wide variation in normal, with some children going several times a day and some babies as often as two dozen times. The consistency of the stool is, however, important.

THE COLOUR OF THE STOOLS isn't usually very important, unless they contain blood.

SHORT BOUTS OF DIARRHOEA are more common in children than the constant diarrhoea which troubles some children. Bouts of diarrhoea are usually the result of **gastroenteritis**, a bowel infection (see *Vomiting*). There may be a temperature and vomiting, and other members of the family may be affected.

GUIDANCE
Dehydration, excess loss of body fluid, is the main danger, although it doesn't often arise from diarrhoea unless there is vomiting too. Nevertheless, small babies may be at risk, and you should check for signs of dehydration (see *Vomiting*) and try to get your baby to **drink** as much as possible.

Clear liquids and juices are fine, or best of all is a salt and sugar mixture from the chemist which replaces lost fluids most efficiently. Don't try to mix salt and sugar in water at home, as the **exact proportions are critical** and an imbalance could be dangerous.

❖   ❖   ❖

Eating should continue as normal while your child has diarrhoea, although dairy products may sometimes prolong the diarrhoea and are probably best avoided. Breast-fed babies should continue to feed as normal.

❖   ❖   ❖

Drugs to slow the diarrhoea are almost always best avoided. Diarrhoea due to an infection is part of the body's response to invading bugs, and helps to flush them out of the bowel. Slowing the diarrhoea with drugs may prevent this, and actually prolong the illness. The drugs certainly won't clear diarrhoea any more quickly. Occasionally they may be useful when it is important temporarily to control diarrhoea in older children, such as during a journey. Paracetamol is useful for fever or pains (see dosage, page 11).

SEE YOUR DOCTOR if diarrhoea lasts more than ten days. Diarrhoea due to an infection may take this long to clear but if it hasn't there may be something else going on. Sometimes the problem is temporary damage to the lining of the bowel which prevents the child from digesting milk; a dairy-free diet for a few weeks usually does the trick.

BLOODY DIARRHOEA should ALWAYS BE SEEN BY A DOCTOR. Some bugs, particularly those that cause food poisoning, may be responsible and may occasionally need treatment with antibiotics. The doctor will rule out other possible causes such as intussusception (a bowel obstruction – see *Crying babies*) or colitis, an inflammation of the bowel.

DIARRHOEA WITH PAIN is common, as the over-active bowel **goes into spasm** producing colicky cramping stomach pains which come and go, usually on the left side. If the pains are occasional, aren't getting worse, your child is fine in between, and his or her abdomen isn't tender when you press it, then you can safely treat the pains with paracetamol (see dosage, page 11) and a hot water bottle.

Otherwise you should CHECK WITH YOUR DOCTOR to rule out rarer possibilities such as appendicitis or intussusception.

DIARRHOEA DUE TO CERTAIN FOODS is quite common in children and sometimes in breast-fed babies because of the food their mothers ear. Spicy foods and large amounts of fruit are common culprits and you should simply cut down the amount.

A child who has diarrhoea after a wide range of food, should SEE THE DOCTOR to check that he or she is absorbing food properly. Some drugs , particularly a course of antibiotics, may set off diarrhoea too.

CONSTANT OR LONGSTANDING DIARRHOEA is likely to be a different problem with different causes. Occasionally, infections are to blame, or milk intolerance as the aftermath of an infection (see above).

LONGSTANDING DIARRHOEA IN BABIES can be quite normal especially if they are breast-fed. Sometimes, too much sugar in the feed can be responsible.

Coeliac disease, where the child's bowel isn't able to digest gluten in wheat and rye products, often causes diarrhoea from the age of around six months when weaning onto wheat products starts. Although hospital tests are needed to confirm the diagnosis, a gluten-free diet provides a cure.

Other diseases, such as cystic fibrosis, may prevent food being absorbed and result in diarrhoea too.

LONGSTANDING DIARRHOEA IN TODDLERS is so common that, when no other cause can be found, it is simply called **toddler diarrhoea**. The cause isn't known, but it is harmless and eventually gets better on its own. Occasionally, anxiety or emotional problems may be responsible.

LONGSTANDING DIARRHOEA STARTING IN OLDER CHILDREN may also be due to anxiety or emotion but can also indicate **colitis**, an inflammation of the bowel.

❖   ❖   ❖   ❖   ❖

GUIDANCE
Some of the above causes may be serious, others not, and as a general rule your child's weight is the best guide. If he or she is gaining weight properly (see *Weight problems*) then it isn't likely that there is anything serious going on. Nevertheless, constant diarrhoea, or a bout of diarrhoea lasting longer than 10 days, should be CHECKED BY YOUR DOCTOR.

❖   ❖   ❖

Treatment of longstanding diarrhoea depends on the cause. If there is no serious or obvious cause then simply waiting for things to improve with time, whilst avoiding any foods that seem to make matters worse, is the best policy.

EYES, RED, SORE OR STICKY

STICKY EYES IN YOUNG AND NEWBORN BABIES are very common. One or both eyes may be affected, often from birth. The whites of the eyes aren't red or sore, but sticky yellow pus builds up which may stick the eyelids together overnight.

Sometimes, in very young babies, an infection is to blame, caught during childbirth. But usually the cause is a **blockage of the tear duct**, the narrow tube that drains tears away from the inside corner of the eye down into the back of the mouth.

GUIDANCE
If the tear duct is blocked, tears can't drain, and will build up in the eye where they become stagnant and sticky.

Although they look a mess, this is harmless, and treatment is simply a matter of continually wiping the sticky pus away with boiled water on cotton wool. Wipe from the inside corner of the eye outwards, and try regularly massaging the inside corner of your baby's eye. This massages the tear duct and will sometimes encourage it to open.

Almost always the blocked tear duct clears itself within a few weeks or months.

❖   ❖   ❖

If there is still a problem after about nine months of age then SEE YOUR DOCTOR, who may arrange for the duct to be cleared by syringing water through it with a fine needle.

❖   ❖   ❖

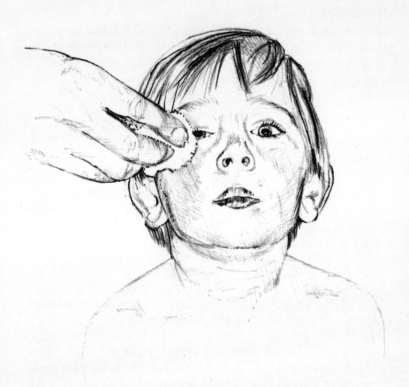

Wipe sticky eyes from the inside corner outwards

Antibiotic eye drops, given by doctors for eye infections, don't usually help, but if the white of your baby's eye becomes red this may indicate an infection and you should SEE YOUR DOCTOR.

STICKY OR RED EYES IN OLDER BABIES AND CHILDREN usually mean **conjunctivitis**, an infection of the transparent lining of the front of the eye. Usually this affects just one eye, although the infection may quickly spread to the other. It starts suddenly, sometimes after a cold, and older children will complain of gritty pain as if they had something in their eye.

81

GUIDANCE
Conjunctivitis is infectious, and can be passed to other children or members of the family through direct contact or through sharing towels and flannels. Your child should be off school, and using his or her own towel.

❖   ❖   ❖

Often the cause is a virus infection, although sometimes an infection with bacteria is responsible.

SEE YOUR DOCTOR. Antibiotic drops or ointment on prescription will help to get rid of bacterial conjunctivitis more quickly. Even without treatment, simply wiping the eye regularly in the way described above (**Sticky eyes in young and newborn babies**), will usually do the trick.

❖   ❖   ❖

SEE YOUR DOCTOR if the conjunctivitis hasn't cleared after five days, in case conjunctivitis isn't to blame.

A RED EYE THAT ISN'T AT ALL STICKY should be CHECKED BY A DOCTOR. Even though conjunctivitis is most likely, he or she will be able to rule out problems such as **uveitis**, an inflammation of the inside of the eye.

ANY DISTURBANCE OF EYESIGHT with a red eye should be CHECKED BY A DOCTOR. Conjunctivitis should never affect the eyesight, although sometimes pus over the front of the eye does make things seem a little blurred.

SOMETHING IN THE EYE usually a speck of dust or dirt, may cause redness and pain.

GUIDANCE
Carefully lift your child's eyelid until you can see the offending object, and remove it with a piece of cotton wool. If you can't do this, then CHECK WITH YOUR DOCTOR.

❖   ❖   ❖

If there is any possibility that a fragment may have **penetrated the eyeball**, for example if the child has been standing close to a grinding wheel, then go STRAIGHT TO CASUALTY.

IF A POKE IN THE EYE causes redness and pain, then CHECK WITH YOUR DOCTOR – there may be a **corneal abrasion**, a graze over the transparent cornea at the front of the eye. This will need careful treatment to avoid the risk of scarring, which could affect your child's sight permanently.

RED ITCHY EYES that come and go, are often caused by an allergy. Usually this will affect both eyes at the same time and, although there is no sticky discharge, the eyes may feel gritty.

Older children may suffer in spring and early summer as part of **hay fever**, an allergy to pollen which usually causes sneezing and an itchy, blocked nose too. Occasionally allergy to other substances is to blame.

GUIDANCE
Keep the child away from situations which you know trigger the symptoms, and use antihistamines from the chemist. SEE YOUR DOCTOR, who will advise about further treatment (see *Hay fever and nose allergies*).

A STYE is an infection of one of the glands in the child's eyelid. It appears quite suddenly as a painful red swelling, usually in the upper eyelid.

The most common glands to be affected are right at the edge of the eyelid, where the eyelashes join the skin. An infection here causes an **external stye**, which is painful for a few days but then disappears on its own without any need for treatment. Sometimes the stye may discharge a small bead of sticky pus; this is quite normal, and simply means that the infection is on its way out.

Less commonly, one of the glands on the inside of the eyelid may become infected. This causes an **internal stye**, usually with more swelling over the whole of the eyelid rather than at just one spot on its edge. Again, it generally settles without treatment, but if the gland remains blocked it may leave a small lump behind. This is a **Meibomian cyst**, a painless lump usually no bigger than a pea, under the upper eyelid.

GUIDANCE
Meibomian cysts are harmless, but if one is obvious or causes discomfort (usually a perpetual feeling that something is in the child's eye), SEE YOUR DOCTOR, as the only treatment is surgical removal. This is a simple and straightforward procedure, under local anaesthetic, in children who are old enough.

❖   ❖   ❖

Treatment for a stye generally means simply waiting for it to go on its own. Warming the eyelid, for example with a flannel soaked in hot water, helps to relieve pain.

F

FAINTING

FAINTS are caused by a sudden drop in blood pressure, to which older children and teenagers seem particularly prone. Faints are quite common in this age group, although parents are understandably terrified at the sight.

A faint may appear out of the blue, although often there are one or more triggers that make it more likely. A virus infection such as a sore throat or flu, strong emotions, a shock, suddenly standing from a sitting or crouching position, a cough, tiredness, or alcohol, can all help to tip the balance.

GUIDANCE
Warning signs usually appear a few seconds before a faint. The child may feel hot and sweaty, and start to lose eyesight with dark spots appearing in front of his or her eyes. There may be a buzzing sound in the ears, followed by a fall and a brief period of unconsciousness. If you are watching, you may notice your child become pale and sweaty just beforehand.

❖   ❖   ❖

Unconsciousness shouldn't last for more than a couple of minutes – it may not occur at all if the child manages to sit or lie down in time once the warning signs start.

HOME TREATMENT
Treatment of fainting is a matter of reassuring your child that there is nothing wrong, and always trying to avoid triggers that may be responsible.

❖   ❖   ❖

If your child is unconscious, then

✦ Lie him or her on one side, with the top arm pulled forward and the top leg bent at the hip and knee, to avoid rolling over.

✦ Support the child's neck and back with a pillow, if necessary, but don't put a pillow under the head.

✦ Make sure that the child's head is lying on the floor with the jaw and tongue pulled forward so that he or she can breathe.

✦ **Don't** try to sit up or stand up a child who is unconscious, as this could interfere with the blood supply to the brain.

✦ **Don't** try to give a drink to an unconscious child as this could cause choking. A sip of water once the child is conscious and sitting up may help.

✦ **Don't** be tempted to offer the child a sip of alcohol; it won't help and could even be dangerous.

✦   ✦   ✦

Your child's pulse will be very slow (60 beats per minute or less) immediately after a faint. This is normal, and in fact helps to confirm that a faint was really to blame.

✦   ✦   ✦

Seeing your child faint can be terrifying, but usually there is no need for anything but reassurance. If there is any doubt that a faint was, in fact, to blame you should SEE YOUR DOCTOR AT ONCE.

SEE YOUR DOCTOR if your child

✦ is under 10 years of age (faints aren't very common in this age group), OR

✦ was unconscious for more than a couple of minutes, OR

- can't remember events that happened immediately before the faint (this may suggest a fit rather than a faint), OR

- passed water, bit his or her tongue or fitted during the faint (see **Fits**). These may suggest a fit although a few twitches during a faint can be quite normal.

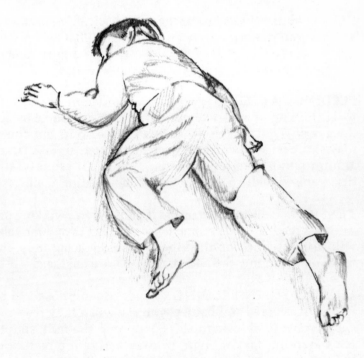

Lie an unconscious child on his or her side

FEEDING PROBLEMS IN BABIES

Feeding your baby is one of the most basic, life-sustaining acts you can perform. So it isn't surprising that babies who don't seem to feed as they should, can cause a great deal of worry and guilt, almost always quite unnecessarily.

FEEDING PATTERNS. All babies are different, and there is no such thing as a normal pattern of feeding. Some babies do choose regular feeds every four or five hours but others may snack on smaller feeds much more often, or take larger amounts but have fewer feeds. Some just seem totally disorganised with no real pattern to their feeding at all.

TENSION. Look out for tension if things aren't working out during a feed. If you become tense or upset then your baby will certainly pick up the vibes – or more accurately, the tension in your muscles and voice – and react to them.

CRYING WHEN FEEDING. Feeds are supposed to be happy occasions, and babies who cry when they feed can cause considerable anguish. Sometimes the milk simply isn't arriving fast enough, or may arrive too fast. Sore nipples, if you are breast-feeding can set off a vicious circle of pain and tension.

Your health visitor is generally the person to advise about feeding techniques.

Some babies seem to suffer colic (see *Colic*).

OCCASIONALLY A SORE MOUTH, usually the result of infection, can make your baby unkeen to feed and cause crying when he or she does. A red inflamed mouth is a clue, maybe with small white fluffy spots (**thrush**, a yeast infection) or painful blisters (infection with the **herpes virus**).

GUIDANCE
Herpes infection usually just has to run its painful course; antifungal drops or gel from your doctor or chemist should help clear thrush.

❖   ❖   ❖

If thrush is the cause and you are breast-feeding, be sure to treat your nipples with cream, as they are sure to be affected.

REGURGITATION is quite normal in babies; they posset, or bring a small amount of feed back up. A little milk goes a long way, and after several possets you may be convinced that there can be nothing left of the original feed. But provided that your baby is putting on weight as he or she should, there is no need to worry. Stained or smelly clothing is the main problem!

GUIDANCE
Posseting may stop after around six months, when your baby starts to sit upright and take solid food; if not it should disappear after one year, once your child starts walking.

❖   ❖   ❖

Your health visitor may suggest powders to thicken the feeds.

RUMINATION is similar, but the child actually seems to regurgitate food deliberately because he or she enjoys the sensation.

VOMITING of large amounts of milk, or of thick lumpy half-digested milk some time after a feed, may not be normal and you should SEE YOUR DOCTOR (see *Vomiting*).

❖   ❖   ❖   ❖   ❖

GUIDANCE
SEE YOUR DOCTOR if your baby

+ isn't gaining weight properly, OR

+ is vomiting, OR

+ has a sore mouth, OR

+ suddenly seems to develop stomach pains.

Your health visitor is often the best person to see for advice about feeding problems.

FEVER AND TEMPERATURE

Young children can develop sudden and alarmingly high temperatures as a result of infections, often virus infections of the nose, throat or ears. A high temperature is part of the body's response to infection, and may help to fight some invading organisms. However, it can also make the child feel unwell, and in susceptible children it increases the risk of fits (febrile convulsions – see *Fits*).

For this reason it is usually advisable to try to bring down a high temperature for the comfort of the child. But don't confuse this with treating the infection itself. Treating a temperature may make the child feel better; it won't shorten the infection, or make it better any more quickly.

GUIDANCE
Usually, it is possible to tell whether your child has a temperature simply by feeling the forehead or chest with your hand. Often this is enough – the exact temperature reading may not be too important, as in itself it doesn't tell you very much about the infection or how ill your child is.

❖   ❖   ❖

Sometimes, however, it is important to use a thermometer to check the exact reading – particularly if your child seems exceptionally hot and won't cool down, or is prone to febrile fits above a certain temperature.

❖   ❖   ❖

Using a thermometer isn't straightforward. First choose your thermometer.

Modern **digital thermometers** display the temperature as

numbers on a tiny display. They are easy to use and read, and work very quickly, but are relatively expensive.

Plastic fever strips placed on a baby's head are useful for a rough assessment of whether or not there is a fever, but aren't as accurate.

❖   ❖   ❖

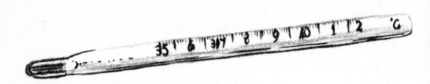

Using a thermometer isn't straightforward

Conventional **mercury column thermometers** are accurate but you must use them correctly. Each one is simply a glass tube containing mercury, with a supply of this stored in a bulb at one end of the tube. As the temperature rises the mercury expands, pushing its way further up the tube. The correct temperature reading is given by the number (marked on the outside of the glass tube) opposite the top of this column of mercury. Modern thermometers show the temperature readings in degrees Celsius (the same as degrees centigrade).

❖   ❖   ❖

Before using a mercury thermometer, hold it by the end furthest away from the bulb and shake it until the top of the mercury column falls well below normal (37 degrees Celsius). Place the whole of the bulb in the child's mouth or armpit (or rectum – see below) and wait for at least two minutes before taking a reading.

❖   ❖   ❖

Where you take your child's temperature makes a great deal of difference to the reading. Older children can hold the bulb in their mouths, under the tongue, and a normal reading would be 37 degrees Celsius. Holding the bulb under the armpit is less accurate, although easier, and will give a reading which is lower by between half and one degree Celsius.

❖   ❖   ❖

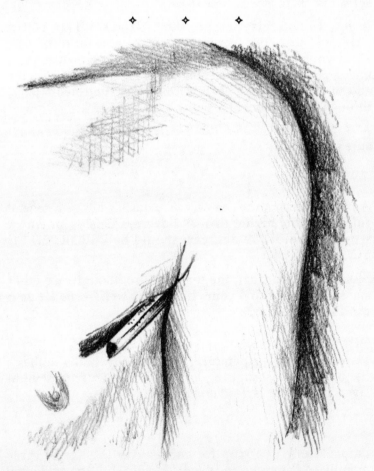

Wait a least two minutes before reading the thermometer

A rectal temperature is most accurate, and is likely to be about half a degree Celsius higher than the mouth temperature.

Taking a rectal temperature means putting the end of the thermometer into your child's rectum, and some doctors used to prefer that parents didn't do this themselves because of the small risk of damage. Recently, however, rectal temperatures have become more popular and most doctors agree that there is very little risk.

If you do use this method, then CHECK WITH YOUR CHEMIST that your thermometer is suitable for rectal use. Hold your baby or toddler firmly face down over your knees, gently separate the opening of the anus and pass the end of the thermometer (lubricated with petroleum jelly) through the anus until the entire bulb is inside.

ASK YOUR DOCTOR OR HEALTH VISITOR if you aren't sure how to do this.

❖ ❖ ❖

A child's temperature can vary very quickly but, as a general rule, **a reading higher than 39.5 degrees Celsius, or which won't go below 39 degrees**, should be REPORTED TO YOUR DOCTOR.

More important than the temperature, though, are other signs suggesting that your child is ill (see *Ill – should your child see the doctor?*).

HOME TREATMENT
To treat a high temperature, take off your child's clothes – the old idea of wrapping a child with a fever in several layers of clothing is dead and buried.

❖ ❖ ❖

Paracetamol, as syrup for babies over the age of three months and as syrup or tablets for older children, will often control a high temperature besides any pain. It works best if you give it regularly, every four hours to a maximum of four times a day (see dosage, page 11).

❖   ❖   ❖

Sponging with tepid water usually works if all else fails. Don't use freezing cold water as this will reduce the circulation to your child's skin, keeping the heat inside the body and actually increasing the temperature. An electric fan, if you have one, directed towards the child, helps.

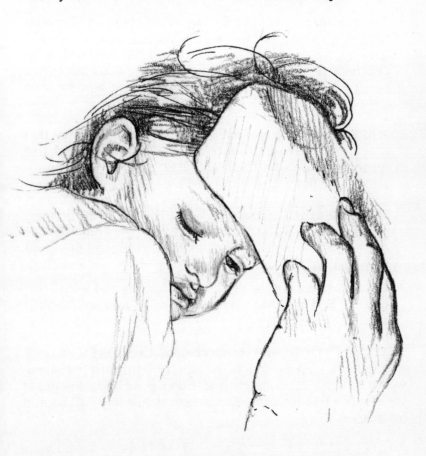

Paracetomol, tepid sponging and a fan all help to cool a fever

FITS

Fits and convulsions mean exactly the same thing. Besides becoming unconscious, the child has uncontrollable movements. Often, these are seen as rhythmical jerking or thrashing movements of arms and legs. The movements may be obvious, or very slight; sometimes children wet themselves or bite their tongues during an attack.

Older children may have the same kind of fit as adults with epilepsy; a sharp cry followed by falling with stiff, rigid muscles, then a jerking fit. Afterwards the child is usually unconscious for several minutes, probably won't remember the fit when he or she wakes, and may be confused for over an hour.

A fit is terrifying to see, and parents are often convinced that their child is dying. In fact, the chances of serious harm during a fit are very small, but it isn't easy to keep this in mind at the time.

FITS IN BABIES are rare, and usually occur in the first few hours of life as a result of lack of oxygen or brain damage during birth. They don't look like fits in older children, and may be difficult to spot.

Older babies may throw their bodies forward with arms outstretched in a kind of spasm. Usually there will be other signs of brain damage.

FITS IN TODDLERS AND YOUNG CHILDREN are very common, because this is the age for **febrile convulsions**. About one child in thirty under the age of five years has at least one febrile convulsion, and the tendency often runs in families.

GUIDANCE
A **febrile convulsion** is a fit that is triggered by a high temperature and, although not all children are susceptible,

these fits are one good reason for trying to control a child's fever (see *Fever and temperature*). Children who have had one febrile convulsion have roughly a one in three risk of having another, and it is particularly important to keep their temperature under control.

❖   ❖   ❖

Children who have had several febrile fits, or whose fits are severe or unusual, may need to take anti-convulsant drugs regularly to prevent more. So SEE YOUR DOCTOR who will sometimes suggest that you keep a supply of **diazepam**. This is a sedative which can be squirted into the rectum of a fitting child to stop a convulsion.

❖   ❖   ❖

Nearly all children with febrile convulsions grow out of them and develop perfectly normally, although a few run the risk of developing epilepsy in later life.

FITS IN OLDER CHILDREN are usually caused by **epilepsy**. This simply means a tendency to fits, which are almost always easily prevented with the right drugs and which the child usually outgrows within ten to twenty years. Nowadays, epilepsy doesn't deserve any of the stigma and strange ideas that still seem to surround it.

Less common forms of epilepsy may not produce classical fits or unconsciousness. **Petit mal epilepsy** causes 'absences' – short periods of loss of attention which may be mistaken for daydreaming. **Temporal lobe epilepsy** may produce fits, but sometimes gives the child strange sensations or odd movements.

❖   ❖   ❖   ❖   ❖

GUIDANCE
SEE A DOCTOR AT ONCE if your child is having, or has had, a fit. Usually a fit is easy to spot, although be sure that

it isn't simply a faint (see *Fainting*) or, in younger children, a breath-holding attack (see *Breath-holding*) or masturbation (see *Masturbation*).

❖ ❖ ❖

Treatment for a fit depends on seeing your doctor. In the meantime, if your child is unconscious, put him or her in the correct position (see *Fainting*).

Don't try to put anything into the mouth to stop your child biting his or her tongue; if this does happen it will be at the beginning of the fit, after which it is too late to do anything but harm by poking into the mouth.

❖ ❖ ❖

Febrile convulsions in children who have had them before, may not need a doctor's immediate attention, but be sure that you have PRECISE INSTRUCTIONS FROM YOUR DOCTOR about what you should do.

FOOT PROBLEMS

Minor deformities of the feet are common in babies and toddlers, but most correct themselves with no treatment.

TALIPES is sometimes still referred to as **a club foot**. Usually the problem is present from birth, and may be caused by pressure on the feet as they were squashed in the womb. In the most common type, the feet are twisted downwards and inwards (**talipes equino-varus**); more rarely they twist in the other direction, upwards and outwards (**talipes calcaneo-valgus**).

GUIDANCE
Talipes should always be CHECKED BY A DOCTOR, although most of the time there is nothing to do and the feet will correct their position with time. Although you should get your doctor's opinion, as a general rule, if your baby has **talipes equino-varus** and you can easily bend the foot upwards so that the toes touch the front of the leg, then there almost certainly isn't a problem.

❖   ❖   ❖

Talipes calcaneo-valgus is more likely to need treatment, and should be watched carefully. Provided the condition is spotted early enough, even if treatment is necessary it is only likely to mean exercises or splinting the foot; surgery is rarely necessary.

FLAT FEET are normal in young children. When an adult stands, the outside edge of the foot rests on the ground while the arch on the inside of the foot rises clear off the ground.
    With flat feet, this inner arch is flattened so that the whole foot rests on the ground.

Babies are born with flat feet, and the inside arch of the foot can take up to six years to develop.

99

GUIDANCE
An easy way to check is to look at your child's bare wet footprint after a bath. If you can see the outline of the whole foot rather than just the outside edge, then the feet are flat.

❖　　　❖　　　❖

In the past, flat feet have been blamed for all manner of problems. In fact they are quite normal in children, and aren't even likely to cause problems in older children or adults.

Special insoles from the chemist, designed to support the inside arch, may help to cut down on shoe wear but they won't make flat feet any less flat.

❖　　　❖　　　❖

Very rarely, flat feet are caused by damage to the nerves controlling the muscles of the foot, leading to pain. **Painful flat feet** are rare in children, and should be CHECKED BY A DOCTOR.

FEET THAT POINT INWARDS are common in children. They may be caused by a deformity of the bones in the foot itself, by twisting of the bones in the lower part of the leg as they grow, or in older children (usually girls) by a twisting of the thigh bone at the hip.

Almost always, they get better without treatment by the age of eight years.

FEET THAT POINT OUTWARDS are common too, usually due to twisting in the other direction of the thigh bone at the hip, and should correct themselves by the age of two.

GUIDANCE
SEE YOUR DOCTOR if toes that turn in or out are actually tripping up your child as he or she walks, or if the toes haven't straightened by the age of eight years (turned in) or two years (turned out).

TALIPES EQUINO-VARUS

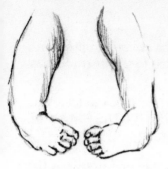

CROOKED TOES

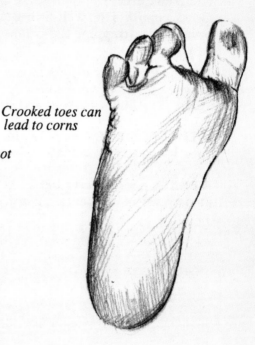

*Crooked toes can
lead to corns*

*Talipes equino-varus may not
need treatment if it is mild*

TALIPES CALCANEO-VALGUS

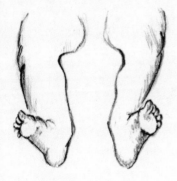

FLAT FEET

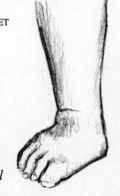

*Talipes calcaneo-valgus will
probably need treatment*

*Flat feet are normal
in young children*

CROOKED TOES can lead to corns and calluses, especially if one toe is jammed over or under the other.

GUIDANCE
Good, comfortable, well-fitting shoes are most important. Sometimes, strapping the crooked toe to the next toe may help.

Usually there isn't any obvious cause for crooked toes, and surgery is rarely necessary. A CHIROPODIST MAY BE ABLE TO HELP with shoes and strapping.

ATHLETE'S FOOT usually affects the area **between the toes**; it is described in *Rashes, long-term*.

VERRUCAS are **warts** that affect the sole of the foot or the underneath of the toes (see *Warts and verrucas*).

FOREIGN OBJECTS

A foreign object is something which is where it shouldn't be. Usually this is the result of an inquisitive child's habit of putting anything that will fit into the nose, ear, vagina or mouth.

Toddlers are usually to blame, which is why it is important to keep a careful eye on children under the age of three years. Although safety regulations mean that toys for this age group don't usually have small parts, pieces of paper, beads, coins, nuts and raisins often find their way where they shouldn't.

FOREIGN OBJECTS IN THE NOSE can be difficult to spot unless your child tell you about them at the time. When the object first enters the nostril it may trigger irritation and sneezing. Afterwards it is quite likely to be forgotten until several days later, when a thick green or yellow smelly discharge, possibly bloodstained, starts to appear from just one nostril.

A runny nose on both sides is likely to mean a cold; a discharge from just one side usually means a foreign object.

GUIDANCE
Treatment will probably involve a doctor, but if your child is old enough to cooperate, you can try blocking the good nostril with your finger, then telling him or her to blow out as hard as possible through the other nostril. If you are lucky this will shoot out the offending object.

If it doesn't work, SEE YOUR DOCTOR. Don't ever try to poke anything into the nostril yourself.

FOREIGN OBJECTS IN THE EAR can also be hard to spot, and may give no symptoms at all. Eventually they will usually produce a sticky or bloody discharge from the ear, and earache.

GUIDANCE
If you know that your child has just put something into his or her ear, then it may be worth running a little **warmed olive oil** into the ear. Sometimes this will float the object out, but never try it unless you are sure that the object has only just gone in.

Never try it if there is a discharge or bleeding from the ear, earache, or the object is a stinging insect. **Never** poke anything into your child's ear, under any circumstances.

❖   ❖   ❖

If olive oil doesn't work or can't be tried, then SEE YOUR DOCTOR with any foreign object in the child's ear.

Removing the object may mean gentle syringing, or pulling out with delicate instruments. For this reason, although some GPs are equipped to perform the procedure, in most areas it is best to take your child STRAIGHT TO CASUALTY.

FOREIGN OBJECTS IN A GIRL'S VAGINA also tend to go unnoticed until a smelly or bloody discharge starts. Unless the object is easy to see and reach, right at the entrance to the vagina, it is best not to try to remove it at all; SEE YOUR DOCTOR.

FOREIGN OBJECTS THAT ARE SWALLOWED are the most common problem. Depending on the age of the child, most objects smaller than a 2p piece will pass through the entire digestive system and out through the other end without problem.

If they do get stuck, this is usually in the **oesophagus** (the gullet, the tube connecting throat and stomach), causing immediate pain and dribbling and preventing the child from swallowing.

Take your child IMMEDIATELY TO CASUALTY if this happens, because the object will probably need to be surgically removed.

OBJECTS THAT ARE SWALLOWED AND DON'T CAUSE SYMPTOMS can usually be safely ignored. Checking or sieving your child's stools for a couple of days, may help to confirm that the object has safely passed.

WHEN DANGEROUS OBJECTS ARE SWALLOWED such as those that are **sharp** or **larger than a 2p piece,** and **batteries, capsules** or **pills,** you should SEE A DOCTOR IMMEDIATELY.

VOMITING, STOMACH PAINS OR CONSTIPATION may suggest the unlikely eventuality that an object has become stuck on its way through the bowel. SEE YOUR DOCTOR IMMEDIATELY if any of these symptoms develop.

FOREIGN OBJECTS THAT ARE BREATHED IN may cause choking if they stick in the throat or windpipe (see *Choking*). Smaller objects that reach further into the lungs may cause no symptoms at first, but carry the risk of chest infections and lung damage.

SEE YOUR DOCTOR if you have any suspicion that your child may have breathed in an object. It will probably need surgical removal with a bronchoscope (a tube passed down the windpipe while the child is anaesthetised).

FOREIGN OBJECTS IN THE EYE – (see *Eyes, red, sore or sticky*).

FORESKIN PROBLEMS

The foreskin is the loose skin covering the glans, the bulb-like end of the **penis**. An adult man's foreskin can normally be pulled right back to expose his glans.

Circumcision means surgical removal of the foreskin. Although there are a few problems for which it does need to be performed, there really don't seem to be any health or hygiene advantages to routine circumcision of a healthy boy.

Religious or cultural beliefs are the most common reason for circumcision of boys in this country. Policies vary from one area of the country to another, but you may well find that cultural circumcision isn't available on the NHS. Your GP should be able to advise you, should you decide to have the operation privately.

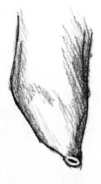 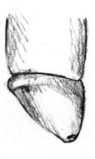

Religious or cultural beliefs are the most common reasons for circumcision

A FORESKIN THAT WON'T PULL BACK is normal in babies and in boys up to the age of five. Never try to force the foreskin back, as this may cause damage. A boy whose foreskin won't pull back after the age of five, should SEE A DOCTOR in case a circumcision is on the cards.

A TINY OPENING IN THE FORESKIN is called a **phimosis**. Normally the opening at the end of the foreskin is quite large. Boys with phimosis may have a very tiny opening indeed, virtually a pinhole. Pressure of urine causes the whole foreskin to swell like a balloon when the child urinates. SEE A DOCTOR. Phimosis needs surgical treatment, usually by circumcision.

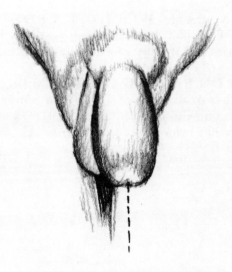

*Phimosis may cause the whole foreskin
to swell when the child urinates*

PAIN IN THE FORESKIN is very common. Sometimes the whole foreskin is red and sore, possibly with a white or yellow discharge. This is **balanitis**, an infection of the foreskin and the glans underneath, and is common especially in boys who are still in nappies.

GUIDANCE
Careful regular cleaning with water, avoiding soap or bath bubbles, usually provides a cure but, if not, SEE YOUR DOCTOR, since antibiotic cream or syrup might do the trick more quickly.

❖   ❖   ❖

Also SEE YOUR DOCTOR if balanitis keeps recurring. The doctor will probably recommend careful washing and hygiene, but may suggest an appointment with a surgeon to consider circumcision if the problem is recurrent and difficult to control.

FORESKIN PAIN WITHOUT REDNESS OR DISCHARGE is also common, and probably indicates minor infections that usually vanish without treatment.

ANY PAIN ON PASSING WATER should be taken seriously. It is probably just a sign of a minor foreskin infection, but you should SEE YOUR DOCTOR to rule out the possibility of a urine infection (see *Urine symptoms*).

HAIR LOSS

Quite often babies and young children lose hair in patches. Although this looks alarming, and is very distressing for a parent to see, the hair virtually always grows back without treatment.

BALD PATCHES IN BABIES are often due to their habit of rolling their head against the mattress or pillow. Babies a few months old seem prone to losing hair anyway, and will rub away a bald patch on one or both sides of their head.

There is no need for treatment, and the hair will grow back normally after the age of one year.

BALD PATCHES IN TODDLERS AND OLDER CHILDREN may have several causes.

Some children **pull at tufts of hair** when they are anxious or insecure; if this becomes a habit it causes one or two bald patches, always in the same place and often covered with fine new hairs that have started to grow back. If you can't persuade your child to stop doing it, then SEE YOUR DOCTOR. Once the hair-pulling stops, the hair should grow back normally.

One or more round bald patches may be due to **alopecia areata** – the name simply means 'bald patches'. The cause is unknown, although it may follow an illness or an emotional shock. Unfortunately, there is no treatment that really seems to work, although usually the bald patches disappear after some months.

Occasionally, **fungus infections** can cause bald patches, usually with itchy, scaly skin, too. There may be rashes on other parts of the body. They can be cured with anti-fungal treatment, so SEE YOUR DOCTOR.

COMPLETE BALDNESS is very rare in children; sometimes it is due to **alopecia totalis**, a severe form of alopecia areata. Some **drugs** that your child is taking may cause hair loss, or occasionally the cause is an inherited abnormality of the hair itself. **Any severe illness** may cause temporary loss of hair.

❖   ❖   ❖   ❖   ❖

GUIDANCE
SEE YOUR DOCTOR if your child has hair loss, to rule out treatable causes such as fungal infection.

❖   ❖   ❖

Avoid tight hair styles that pull on the hairs.

❖   ❖   ❖

Most of the time there isn't anything else that your doctor can offer, except reassurance that most of these conditions do clear up with time.

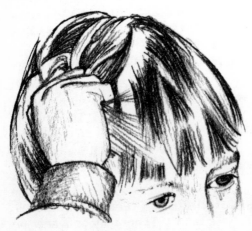

A habit of hair pulling can cause a bald patch

HAY FEVER AND NOSE ALLERGIES

Although hay fever is uncommon in babies and toddlers it is quite common in older children. Hay fever means allergy to pollen, usually grass pollen which is in the air during May and early June.

Symptoms occurring earlier or later in the year may be caused by allergy to other substances, such as tree pollen or mould.

Symptoms all the year round may suggest allergy to house dust or pets.

THE SYMPTOMS OF HAY FEVER are sneezing, a watery runny or blocked nose, itchy watery eyes which may look quite red, and itching of the nose and sometimes throat too.

GUIDANCE
The cause of the allergy is usually possible to identify with time. Symptoms which only occur in the spring and early summer are likely to be due to hay fever. Symptoms all the year round, but which are worse first thing in the morning, suggest house dust allergy.

❖   ❖   ❖

A child can suddenly develop an allergy to a pet which has been in the house for years and, if the symptoms seem to improve when the child is out of the house, then suspect the pet. Don't just remove the pet temporarily to see if there is an improvement; cat and dog hairs cling to carpets and furniture, and may trigger allergy for weeks after the animal has gone.

Symptoms which improve out of a house that doesn't

contain a pet, may suggest house dust allergy, or mould allergy – if there is damp.

❖　　　❖　　　❖

Tests from the doctor aren't likely to help much in pinpointing the cause of the allergy, and your doctor probably won't suggest any.

Trial and error, and careful detective work, are much more reliable.

HOME TREATMENT
Treatment, means removing whatever is triggering the allergy, if possible. Children with hay fever may need to stay indoors on bright spring days. Listen to the radio for details of the pollen count.

❖　　　❖　　　❖

Antihistamine tablets or syrup help to control the symptoms if your child takes them regularly. They are quite safe and are available from the chemist without prescription. Older antihistamines cause drowsiness; ask your chemist for one of the newer types, which don't.

DOCTOR'S TREATMENT
SEE YOUR DOCTOR if these aren't enough to keep the symptoms under control. The doctor may prescribe eye drops and a nasal spray to reduce the allergic reaction.

Occasionally for severe hay fever in older children who are facing an important event such as an exam, the doctor may suggest **steroid tablets**. These are powerful and effective, and quite safe if used in a short course as prescribed.

❖　　　❖　　　❖

Treatment will usually control the symptoms very well. It isn't possible actually to cure hay fever, although a child will normally grow out of it within ten to twenty years.

✧   ✧   ✧

Injections to desensitise children, by injecting larger and larger amounts of pollen until they could tolerate it without a reaction, were once popular but are very rarely given now. They can be dangerous, and several people have died from them – although nobody has ever died from hay fever.

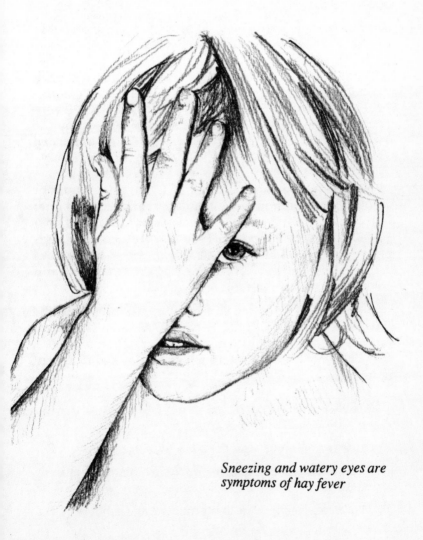

Sneezing and watery eyes are symptoms of hay fever

HEAD INJURIES

Sometimes, even a minor knock on a child's head may produce symptoms that seem quite alarming, whereas more serious injury may produce very few symptoms at first. Knowing what to look for helps you to spot injuries that need a doctor's attention.

Boys are more prone to head injuries than girls, probably because of their more boisterous behaviour.

BLEEDING FROM THE CHILD'S SCALP doesn't really tell you much about the severity of the injury or its possible effects on the brain. The blood supply to the scalp is very good, and even small cuts may bleed profusely. Stop the bleeding and clean and inspect the cut (see *Cuts, scrapes and bruises*). TAKE YOUR CHILD TO CASUALTY if necessary.

CONCUSSION means bruising of the brain, and minor degrees of concussion are common in children even after slight blows to the head. Minor concussion may send your child white and pale, and he or she may feel sick and sleepy with a headache. This should all recover within two or three hours, and needs no treatment apart from rest and paracetamol for pain (see dosage, page 11).

Any possibility of more serious concussion should be CHECKED BY A DOCTOR STRAIGHT AWAY. This might indicate serious brain bruising, or the formation of a blood clot on the surface of the brain which might need treatment by surgery.

GUIDANCE
SEE YOUR DOCTOR if your child

❖   was unconscious after the blow, however briefly, OR

❖   can't remember the blow or the events just before it, OR

❖   isn't completely back to normal within six hours, OR

❖ vomits (apart from once, immediately after the injury), OR

❖ is increasingly drowsy and difficult to wake, OR

❖ has a headache which is getting worse, OR

❖ has crossed eyes or blurred or double vision, OR

❖ has a bloodstained discharge from nose or ear (possible leak of brain fluid, a sign of serious injury), OR IF

❖ the **fontanelle** (the soft spot on the top of a baby's head) is tense and bulging.

Some children may seem pale and under the weather for several days following a minor blow, but recover fully in the end.

PREVENTION
Prevention of head injuries includes: using stair gates around the house; encouraging crash helmets for children on cycles, roller skates or skateboards; and keeping a careful eye on young children all the time, but especially around playgrounds and outdoors.

Your health visitor should be able to give you more advice.

HEAD LICE

Head lice affect one in ten children from all walks of life. No one is immune, but sometimes the lice do seem to prefer one person rather than another; the reason for this is often a mystery. Dirty hair isn't a cause and in fact, if anything, the lice seem to prefer clean hair.

The lice are tiny flat insects about three or four millimetres in length. They live in human hair, and can't live on other parts of the body or on animals.

SYMPTOMS OF HEAD LICE are usually an itchy scalp, particularly at the sides and at the back; and if you look carefully at the hair behind your child's ears and over his or her neck, you may see nits.

Nits are eggs laid by the lice; usually they are firmly stuck to the hair shaft at its base where it joins the scalp. The nits are white or pinkish and may look like flakes of dandruff. The difference is easy to spot because nits, unlike dandruff, won't fall off when the hair is shaken.

Spotting the lice themselves is usually impossible, because they scurry out of the way when you start to explore your child's hair.

Spread of head lice is caused by direct contact with someone who is infested, or by sharing combs, hairbrushes or hats.

HOME TREATMENT
Treatment is usually straightforward, with a cream, lotion or shampoo available from your chemist or on prescription from your doctor. Some shampoos are designed to prevent head lice and aren't strong enough actually to treat them so, if you use a shampoo, make sure that your chemist knows which you need.

❖   ❖   ❖

It is important that every member of the family is treated at the same time – otherwise it is quite possible for some members to be infested without any symptoms at all, and to pass the lice straight back again. Use a fine comb (a **nit comb**, available from your chemist) to remove lice and nits from your child's hair while this is wet. Treatment usually works well.

DOCTOR'S TREATMENT
Lice that keep coming back are likely to mean that your child is being reinfested, often at school. SEE YOUR DOCTOR in this case. Occasionally lice are resistant to the older preparations such as malathion or carbaryl, and your doctor may suggest treatment with a newer preparation such as **pyrethrin**.

❖   ❖   ❖

Be prepared to follow your doctor's or chemist's advice on treatment.

Many areas of the country have a local policy stating which preparation should be used. This is to reduce the danger of lice developing resistance to several preparations at once. If local lice start to develop resistance to the recommended preparation, another is chosen.

HEARING PROBLEMS

Complete or severe deafness is rare in children, but partial deafness – which may interfere with school and the development of proper speech – is common. It probably affects around ten per cent of children in this country, at one time or another.

HEARING PROBLEMS IN BABIES can be hard to spot. After birth, your baby should jump and be startled by a loud noise, by blinking or opening his or her eyes. By about four weeks, the baby should become quiet and still to a loud sound; and by three months, should smile and quieten at the sound of your voice and start to turn towards a sound coming from the side.

By six months, your baby should turn to your voice or to very quiet noises coming from the side; and by nine months, should listen carefully to familiar sounds, should babble and look around for a sound made out of sight. By twelve months, most babies will respond to their own name and other words.

SEE YOUR DOCTOR OR HEALTH VISITOR if you aren't sure about any of the above, or if you have any other reason to think that your baby isn't hearing properly.

HEARING PROBLEMS IN TODDLERS AND YOUNG CHILDREN may be more obvious, although slight deafness that comes and goes may be hard to pin down. Your child's speech is the best guide; if he or she is saying single words clearly and understandably around the age of one year, putting words together by the age of two years, and making understandable sentences at three years, then a significant hearing problem is unlikely.

Again, you should CHECK WITH YOUR DOCTOR OR HEALTH VISITOR if you have any doubt about your child's ability to hear slight sounds and to catch everything you say.

HEARING PROBLEMS IN OLDER CHILDREN may not affect their speech. Sometimes the first sign is a deterioration in a child's behaviour and school work. The child may ask for the television to be turned up, or constantly ask adults to repeat themselves. This can be normal behaviour in all children, but use common sense and be especially suspicious if your child seems to understand you better when he or she can see your face – he or she may be partly lip-reading.

GUIDANCE
The most common cause of deafness in children is **serous otitis media** (glue ear). This means there is fluid in the middle ear cavity, the part of the ear just behind the ear drum which is normally filled with air. The fluid prevents sounds from being carried across the middle ear to nerves, which then carry it to the brain.

Normally, middle ear fluid drains away through the **eustachian tube**, connecting the middle ear cavity to the back of the throat. Glue ear arises when the eustachian tube can't drain properly. This may happen because of repeated colds or middle ear infections; enlarged adenoid glands in the back of the throat; allergy; or a combination of factors (see *Pain or discharge in the ear*).

The amount of fluid in the middle ear may vary greatly, even from one day to the next, so a child whose hearing seems to vary from day to day may have a genuine problem.

❖　　　❖　　　❖

Less common causes of deafness in children include wax or foreign objects in the ear (see *Foreign objects*), or damage to the nerve-carrying impulses from the ear to the brain as a side effect of some drugs.

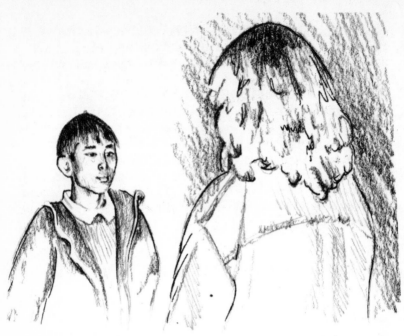

A child who studies your face as you talk may be partly lip-reading

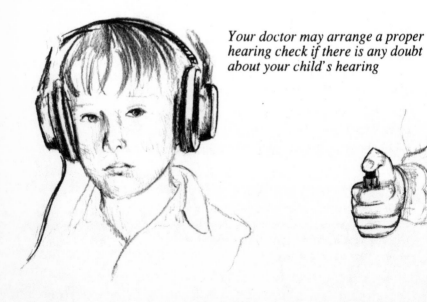

Your doctor may arrange a proper hearing check if there is any doubt about your child's hearing

Brain damage is sometimes responsible. This may be: from infections such as meningitis; from infections such as rubella (German measles) caught by the mother before the baby is born; from a head injury; from damage during birth; or from severe jaundice after birth. Usually, these cause more severe and permanent deafness.

❖   ❖   ❖

Treatment of deafness means first spotting it. If you have any doubts about your child's hearing, then CHECK WITH YOUR DOCTOR OR HEALTH VISITOR, who may arrange a proper hearing check.

❖   ❖   ❖

Routine hearing tests are an important part of the checks performed on all children at around six weeks, six to nine months, two to two-and-a-half years and three years of age. The exact ages vary from one area of the country to another.

DOCTOR'S TREATMENT
The doctor's treatment of **glue ear** may involve time – the problem usually cures itself in the end – together with antibiotics, treatments for allergy, or surgery to remove adenoid glands that are blocking the eustachian tube or to put tubes or grommets into the ear drum. These provide an opening in the ear drum, connecting the middle ear cavity with the outside. This brings the pressure in the middle ear back to normal, and allows any fluid to drain properly.

❖   ❖   ❖

More severe deafness may need other treatment, including hearing aids and special schools.

HYPERACTIVITY

A few children are so excessively active and energetic that they may be a positive danger to themselves, as well as being unable to learn or concentrate on virtually anything.

There is no precise medical definition of hyperactivity, which sometimes makes the diagnosis a matter of opinion. In America, up to one in ten children are described as hyperactive; in this country doctors are stricter about the diagnosis, and the figure is more likely to be around one child in a thousand.

Often, children have more energy than their parents and may, quite normally, be on the go all day and sometimes at night too. A truly hyperactive child is different, and his or her behaviour usually manages to impress everyone in the room immediately.

HYPERACTIVE CHILDREN are positively bursting with activity all day, and don't seem to need much sleep at night.

Their concentration is very poor, and they won't settle to one task for more than a few seconds before being distracted by something else. Sitting quietly with the child to read a book or watch TV is impossible.

GUIDANCE
Diagnosing hyperactivity can be very difficult, and most very active children aren't really hyperactive. One clue may be slow development. Hyperactive children have such poor concentration that their speech and reading skills may lag behind, whereas normal (but very active) children develop on time.

If you have any doubts, ASK YOUR DOCTOR OR HEALTH VISITOR, who will be able to arrange an expert assessment if necessary.

❖   ❖   ❖

The cause of hyperactivity isn't known, and there may be different causes in different children. Slight brain damage during birth is one possibility.

Another possibility is artificial colourings in food and drink. Some doctors think that these trigger hyperactivity in susceptible children, but other doctors disagree. If you do suspect that food additives affect your child's behaviour it is best to make changes only after CHECKING WITH YOUR DOCTOR OR HEALTH VISITOR, and possibly AFTER CONSULTING A DIETICIAN.

❖ ❖ ❖

Treatment of hyperactivity usually means seeing a specialist. Drugs don't often help much although, strangely enough, stimulants – which cause excitation and activity in adults – actually seem to quieten some hyperactive children.

A special school may be necessary, as hyperactive children have such poor concentration that they tend to do badly in class.

ILL – SHOULD YOUR CHILD SEE THE DOCTOR?

In this section a few clues and guidelines are suggested to help you decide whether an illness is potentially serious, and whether you should see a doctor. However, it is no substitute for your experience and instinct.

You know your child better than anyone else, and you know his or her reactions to illness. You are in the best position to judge how ill your child really is. If your child **just seems very unwell**, whatever the cause and whether or not any of the signs in this chapter are present, then SEE YOUR DOCTOR.

ILLNESS IN BABIES often doesn't give many clues. The baby simply seems generally miserable, with poor feeding, crying, maybe vomiting or diarrhoea. SEE YOUR DOCTOR with any of the following.

- ✤ Any unexplained illness lasting more than 12 hours.

- ✤ Unexplained constant crying lasting more than one hour, or a cry which sounds very different from normal.

- ✤ Vomiting lasting more than 12 hours.

- ✤ Diarrhoea containing blood.

- ✤ A baby who feels floppier than normal.

◆ A fontanelle (the soft spot on the top of the baby's head) which has sunken (possibly dehydration) or is tense and bulging (possibly meningitis). It pays to get used to the way your baby's fontanelle normally feels, to help spot any difference.

◆ A baby who holds the head back, or won't let you move the head (possible meningitis).

◆ Signs of dehydration (see *Vomiting*).

◆ Difficult breathing, especially with a noise (see *Breathing, noisy or difficult*) or sucking in of the skin between and underneath the ribs as the child breathes.

◆ Rapid breathing (over 60 breaths per minute when the baby is awake, or over 40 per minute when asleep).

◆ Blue colour around the face and lips (blue hands and feet may be normal in babies).

◆ Skin colour change – excessively pale, or yellow (see *Jaundice*).

ILLNESS IN TODDLERS AND OLDER CHILDREN is often easier to pinpoint. Useful warning signs that you should SEE YOUR DOCTOR include any of the following.

◆ Diarrhoea containing blood.

◆ Confusion (the child doesn't know where he or she is, or what day it is. A very high temperature may also trigger delirium, when the child see things that aren't there).

◆ A child whom you can't keep awake or who doesn't seem fully conscious.

◆ An unexplained pain in the head, chest or abdomen that is getting worse after a couple of hours (see *Pain in the head; Pain in the chest; Pain in the abdomen, sudden*).

◆ An unusually high temperature (see *Fever and temperature*).

❖   Signs of dehydration (see *Vomiting*).

❖   A stiff painful neck that prevents the child from touching the chest with his or her chin (possibility of meningitis – see *Pain in the head*).

❖   A rash on the body made of small, flat purple blotches (possibility of meningitis – see *Rashes, sudden*).

❖   Swelling around the eyes and mouth (possible allergic reaction).

❖   Difficult or rapid breathing (over 35 breaths per minute at the age of five years), especially if the skin between and under the ribs becomes sucked in with each breath (see *Breathing, noisy or difficult*).

❖   Blue colour around the lips.

❖   A yellow colour to the skin (see *Jaundice*).

❖   ❖   ❖   ❖   ❖

Most important of all: SEE A DOCTOR IMMEDIATELY if you simply **feel** that your child really is **ILL**.

IMMUNISATION REACTIONS

Babies in this country should receive jabs to protect against diphtheria, tetanus, pertussis (whooping cough) and Hib (Haemophilus influenzae B – an important cause of meningitis), together with vaccine against polio given by mouth. A course of three jabs is needed, given at the ages of two, three and four months.

Older children should have the MMR jab protecting against measles, mumps and rubella (German measles) between the ages of 12 and 15 months. A pre-school booster against diphtheria, tetanus and polio is usually given around three-and-a-half years, after which the child should have booster jabs against tetanus every 10 years, for life.

SERIOUS REACTIONS TO THESE VACCINES are very rare indeed. The measles and whooping cough vaccines were once thought to cause (but rarely) brain damage. Nowadays, most doctors think that this doesn't happen at all.

Older types of MMR vaccine carried the risk of meningitis, an infection around the brain, but the risk is much less with the newer types – probably around one in three hundred thousand. Usually this form of meningitis is mild with no serious effects.

Very rarely, MMR vaccine may reduce the number of platelets in the child's blood. Platelets help the blood to clot, and a low platelet count may cause bruising or a rash of flat purple blotches; usually the problem gets better without any treatment, but should be CHECKED WITH THE DOCTOR.

Very rarely – about one in two million cases – someone who isn't immunised against polio may catch the disease from a baby who has recently had the vaccine. This underlines the importance of everyone being protected.

MORE COMMON REACTIONS TO THE VACCINES are usually very mild. A red area of skin around where the jab was given is quite common, and should disappear within a few days. SEE YOUR DOCTOR if the redness spreads most of the way around your child's leg or arm.

Sometimes a small hard lump is left behind; this is quite normal and should disappear in time, although this might take several months.

HIGH TEMPERATURE is quite likely, usually within a day or two of diphtheria/tetanus/pertussis (DTP) vaccine but around a week after MMR. Crying and high-pitched screaming occasionally follow DTP vaccine; although upsetting, it doesn't last long and doesn't mean that anything is wrong.

SWELLING OF THE PAROTID GLAND. Around one in a hundred children will develop swelling of this gland, under the ear, which makes saliva, after the MMR jab. The swelling may affect one or both sides, and usually happens around three weeks after the jab. The swelling gradually disappears without any treatment.

A FINE RASH may appear over the body about a week after MMR. This is normal, doesn't mean that the child is infectious, and will disappear within a few days.

JOINT PAINS. Occasionally, children may develop joint pains several weeks after MMR, usually in their arms or legs. The pains are mild, soon disappear, and will improve with paracetamol (see dosage, page 11) if necessary.

❖   ❖   ❖   ❖   ❖

GUIDANCE
Treatment of immunisation reactions usually means simply waiting.

Paracetamol is good to treat high temperatures, even in babies of two months. If your child has had high temperatures with previous jabs, or if it is particularly important to avoid high temperatures (for example because of febrile convulsions in the past – see *Fits*) then it is best to give paracetamol regularly, to prevent any fever (see dosage, page 11)

❖   ❖   ❖

Overall, these immunisations are extremely safe, unlike the diseases that they are designed to protect against. Your doctor or health visitor will be happy to discuss any doubts about vaccination that you may have.

ITCHING ANUS

THREADWORMS are the most common cause of an itchy bottom in children. They are tiny, thin white worms one centimetre or so in length, and look like a short piece of white thread.

Threadworms live just inside a child's anus, but come out onto the skin outside to lay their eggs. Usually they do this at night, which explains why the itching they cause is generally much worse at night. They may look alarming if you catch sight of them, but they are completely harmless and the only symptom they cause is an itchy bottom.

Scratching his or her bottom lodges the eggs under the child's fingernails. Contact with other children, or playing with their food, will then pass the eggs on to someone else; the eggs hatch in the new child's bowel after a couple of weeks, and the cycle continues.

Children, with their less than hygienic habits, are usually affected and threadworms are very common in school- and nursery-aged children.

GUIDANCE
Diagnosing threadworms usually means an itchy bottom, especially at night. Occasionally you may see the worms themselves in your child's stool – you can tell them from pieces of thread or tissue paper because they wriggle. If more than one person in the family has an itchy bottom at the same time, then the diagnosis of threadworms is almost certain.

❖   ❖   ❖

Usually there isn't any need to confirm the diagnosis, but if necessary your doctor can apply a piece of sticky tape to your child's bottom and arrange for the tape to be examined under a microscope. Any eggs will stick to the tape and be seen through the microscope.

❖   ❖   ❖

Treating threadworms is usually easy, with medicine bought from your chemist or on prescription from your doctor. It is important to treat everyone in the family, in case they are carrying the worms with no symptoms. CHECK WITH YOUR DOCTOR if you are pregnant, or if your child is under one year old.

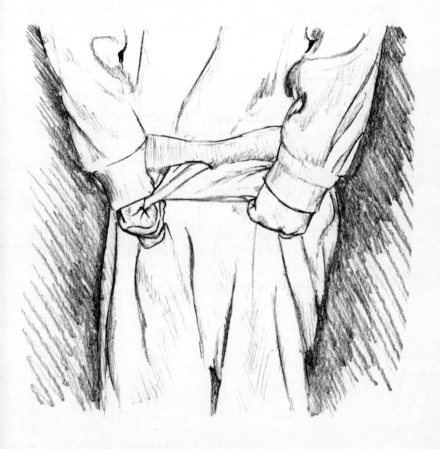

An itchy bottom is often the only symptom of thread worms

131

❖   ❖   ❖

Cut your child's fingernails short, to reduce the chances of eggs lodging underneath, and make sure that the nails are scrubbed after using the loo. Pyjama trousers rather than nighties will help to stop little girls scratching their bottoms in their sleep.

OTHER CAUSES OF AN ITCHY BOTTOM are less common in children. Sometimes **dermatitis**, a patch of inflamed dry skin, is to blame – particularly if the child is prone to dry sensitive skin.

Keep the anus clean and dry, avoid soap or bath bubbles and use a moisturising or steroid cream such as hydrocortisone from your doctor.

Infections, usually with fungus, can cause itching, too, and can be cured with an anti-fungal cream from your doctor or chemist.

Occasionally the cause can't be found.

❖   ❖   ❖   ❖   ❖

SEE YOUR DOCTOR to confirm the diagnosis if your child's itchy bottom doesn't get better after threadworm treatment, or if there is a rash around the anus (suggesting dermatitis or fungal infection).

ITCHING ANYWHERE

Itching is a common problem and, although there are dozens of possible causes, there are usually different clues to help the diagnosis.

ITCHY SPOTS are usually due to allergy, insect bites or infections such as chickenpox (see *Spots, itchy*).

AN ITCHY RASH is most likely to suggest dermatitis or a fungus infection, or an allergy (see *Rashes, sudden*). Some children develop an itchy sweat rash in the heat, or whenever their skin is in contact with wool or nylon.

HOME TREATMENT
Avoiding these triggers, keeping the skin clean and dry without soap or bubbles, and using steroid cream from the doctor as necessary, will usually provide a cure.

URTICARIA (**hives**, or so-called **nettle rash**) is one form of itchy rash which is usually easy to identify. It is most common under the age of five years, and appears as itchy, white weals and red blotches which keep appearing and disappearing again very quickly – over a period of hours. No other rash comes and goes as quickly as this.

Often there is no obvious cause, but allergy to a food or drug is sometimes to blame. Sometimes emotional stress or a virus infection may be the trigger.

HOME TREATMENT
Antihistamine syrup or tablets, available from the chemist, is usually the best treatment. Older types of antihistamine cause drowsiness; the newer drugs don't make the child drowsy, but may be less effective for itching.

❖   ❖   ❖

If antihistamines don't work, if there is swelling around your child's mouth or eyes (suggesting more serious allergy), or if the urticaria doesn't disappear within a few days, SEE YOUR DOCTOR.

SCALP ITCHING may be caused by head lice, although there are other causes (see *Head lice* and *Cradle cap and dandruff*).

VERY INTENSE ITCHING, USUALLY IN SKIN CREASES such as armpits, wrists and between the fingers, may be caused by scabies. **Scabies** is a mite which burrows under the skin; it is passed on by direct contact with an infested person. Usually you can see tiny spots where the mites have entered the skin. SEE YOUR DOCTOR, who will look carefully for burrows, the tracks made by the mites as they burrow under the skin, but these can be hard to see.

Other members of the family may be affected too.

HOME TREATMENT
Scabies causes very severe itching, especially at night (in medieval days it was known simply as 'The Itch'). Fortunately, treatment has improved since those days, and a single application of lotion should do the trick.

You should SEE YOUR DOCTOR FIRST to confirm the diagnosis, and follow his or her instructions carefully about applying the lotion.

ITCHING ALL OVER WITHOUT ANY RASH OR SPOTS AT ALL is much less common, and it may be difficult to find the cause.

GUIDANCE
If it starts suddenly, an allergy or infection may be to blame.

Several drugs can cause itching, and you should CHECK WITH YOUR DOCTOR about any that your child is taking.

Stress or emotional problems are sometimes to blame.

❖   ❖   ❖

More rarely, diseases such as jaundice (see *Jaundice*), leukaemia, lymphoma or diabetes may be the cause.

If there is no obvious cause for the itching, then you should SEE YOUR DOCTOR if it carries on for more than one day. In the meantime, try treatment with antihistamines (see **Urticaria**, above).

JAUNDICE

Jaundice means a yellow colour to the skin caused by a build-up of **bilirubin**. Bilirubin is a waste product formed when old, worn-out red blood cells are destroyed to make way for new cells.

Normally, bilirubin is efficiently disposed of by the liver. But if there is more bilirubin than the liver can handle, or if the liver is damaged and can't cope with the normal amount, then bilirubin will build up and jaundice results.

GUIDANCE
The diagnosis of jaundice is usually obvious from the child's yellow colour; yellowing of the whites of the eyes is the first sign.

❖　　　❖　　　❖

Occasionally jaundice isn't to blame. Some drugs, or large amounts of carrots or tomatoes, may occasionally turn the skin yellow, although not the whites of the eyes.

❖　　　❖　　　❖

Spotting jaundice is, however, only the first step; it is essential to find the cause.

JAUNDICE IN NEWBORN BABIES is very common in the first few days of life, and probably affects about half of all babies in this country, to some extent. The problem is that the tiny baby's liver isn't yet fully equipped to handle bilirubin. However, the liver develops quickly, and this kind of jaundice – known as **physiological jaundice** – usually starts to improve after the third or fourth day.

GUIDANCE
The danger is that, if the level of bilirubin in the baby's blood rises too high, fits and brain damage may result. Normally this isn't a problem with physiological jaundice, although your DOCTOR OR MIDWIFE WILL KEEP A CHECK on the bilirubin level, if necessary. Usually this means analysing a blood sample taken from a heel prick.

❖   ❖   ❖

Treatment of physiological jaundice isn't usually necessary, although your baby should drink as much fluid as possible, to dilute the bilirubin in the blood. This isn't as easy as it sounds as one side-effect of jaundice is to make the baby drowsy, and often too sleepy to be interested in a drink.

If necessary, **phototherapy** – shining a blue light onto the baby's skin – helps to destroy the bilirubin in the skin. Leaving your baby exposed by a sunny window may help too.

JAUNDICE THAT ISN'T PHYSIOLOGICAL is rarer, but may be more serious. Rhesus disease, where the baby's red blood cells are destroyed by the mother's blood in the womb, is one possibility. Others include infection or liver abnormalities.

❖   ❖   ❖   ❖   ❖

GUIDANCE
SEE YOUR DOCTOR if jaundice develops within 24 hours of birth – physiological jaundice never does this. Jaundice lasting longer than 10 days should be checked, too; physiological jaundice usually disappears by this time. Occasionally it may quite normally last longer, especially in breast-feeding babies (probably because of the effect on the baby's liver of hormones in the breast milk).

❖   ❖   ❖

If your baby is very drowsy, doesn't want to feed, seems ill (see *Ill – should your child see the doctor?*), or the jaundice is getting worse after the third day of life, then CHECK WITH THE DOCTOR, too.

JAUNDICE IN OLDER CHILDREN usually means **infectious hepatitis**. This is caused by a virus which infects the liver and, as the name suggests, it is infectious. Usually, children catch it by contact with, or eating food prepared by, someone who is infected. In developing countries, the virus may be present in drinking water.

Jaundice usually appears after about a week of mysterious sickness, loss of appetite, stomach pains and feeling generally unwell. There may be pain under the lower part of the rib-cage at the front, from the liver swelling. The child's stools may turn pale and the urine dark.

GUIDANCE
SEE YOUR DOCTOR. The jaundice may be itchy, and usually fades after a week or two, but may occasionally last for weeks or even months. Most children feel weak and tired for some time, and should expect to be off school for between two and six weeks.

❖   ❖   ❖

Treatment of infectious hepatitis simply involves keeping your child comfortable, drinking plenty, and in bed for the first few days when the symptoms are worst.

❖   ❖   ❖

Those in contact with the child for the first couple of weeks should wash their hands thoroughly afterwards.

OTHER CAUSES OF JAUNDICE IN OLDER CHILDREN are more rare. Some drugs, and even solvent abuse, can affect the liver and cause jaundice. Other infections, such as glandular fever, may occasionally be to blame.

Inherited conditions where the red blood cells are unusually fragile, and become destroyed faster than the liver can cope with the bilirubin they release, include elliptocytosis, sickle cell (in children of Afro-Caribbean descent) and thalassaemia (in children of Mediterranean descent).

❖   ❖   ❖   ❖   ❖

SEE YOUR DOCTOR if you suspect that your child has developed jaundice, to confirm the diagnosis and to find the cause.

KNOCK KNEES

Just as bow legs are so common as to be normal in toddlers, knock knees probably affect around three-quarters of older children in this country, particularly between the ages of three and five years.

GUIDANCE
Diagnosis of knock knees is usually easy. When the child stands with the legs straight and the knees touching, the lower part of the legs splay outwards so that the ankles don't touch.

❖   ❖   ❖

The cause of knock knees is usually simply that the child is developing quite normally. Very rarely, an injury, or a disease such as rickets which softens the bones, is responsible.

❖   ❖   ❖

Treatment is usually completely unnecessary; the condition is normal and the legs will straighten within a few years.

Very rarely, in severe cases after the age of 10 years, surgery is involved. This may mean breaking the femur (the bone in the thigh) or the tibia (the main bone in the lower leg) and removing a wedge of bone to straighten the leg. Some surgeons recommend wearing wedges in the shoes to try to straighten the bones without surgery, but most doctors nowadays don't believe that this works.

❖   ❖   ❖

SEE YOUR DOCTOR if

❖ your child has very obvious knock knees after the age
  of 10 years, OR

❖ only one knee is affected, OR

❖ the distance between the inside of the ankles, when the
  child stands up straight, is more than 10 centimetres.

Otherwise you should be able to wait confidently for the
condition to get better on its own.

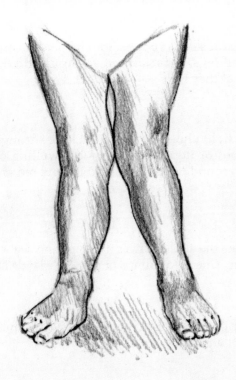

*See your doctor if there is more than 10 cm
between the inside of your child's ankles
when standing straight*

LIMPING

The cause of a child's limping is usually obvious if he or she has had a recent knock or fall. Sometimes, especially with younger children, it isn't possible to be so sure and in this case limping should always be taken seriously.

GUIDANCE
Finding the cause of a sudden limp involves a careful look at the feet and legs, especially in young children who can't explain what they feel.

❖　　　❖　　　❖

Check for tight shoes, or a nail sticking through the sole; infected toes or ingrowing toenails; swelling or bruising especially around the ankle and knee; any red areas or sore spots.

❖　　　❖　　　❖

Gently move the ankles, knees and hips and see whether this causes pain. Check for lumps or swollen glands in the groin.

❖　　　❖　　　❖

See if your child is anxious or upset – stress and emotions can occasionally cause limping.

❖　　　❖　　　❖

If there is no obvious cause that you can treat yourself, then try putting your child to bed. If he or she is still limping for no obvious reason by the next day, then SEE YOUR DOCTOR.

❖   ❖   ❖

Bruising or injury is the most common cause of limping. Active, older children often have minor muscle tears and sprains which should clear with time and rest.

PAIN IN THE HIP may cause limping, and should always be taken seriously. Children aged between five and ten years may be suffering from **Perthe's disease**. Here, the blood supply to the top of the thigh bone which forms part of the hip joint (the ball in the ball and socket joint) is damaged, although no one knows why.

This causes hip pain and a limp; sometimes the child actually feels the pain in the knee rather than the hip. Usually, Perthe's disease recovers without treatment, although arthritis much later in life is a slight risk, and you should SEE YOUR DOCTOR for regular X-ray checks on the state of the hip joint.

HIP PAIN IN OLDER CHILDREN AND ADOLESCENTS between 10 and 20 years may suggest a **slipped epiphysis**.

Adults' bones are all in one piece; childrens' bones are actually formed from two or more pieces joined by a layer of cartilage, to allow for growth. One such layer of cartilage joins the top of the thigh bone, which forms the ball of a ball and socket joint, to the rest of the thigh bone.

This layer must take most of the weight of the child's body, and occasionally this will be more than the cartilage can bear. The ball at the top of the thigh bone slips downwards, gradually producing pain and a limp. As with other causes of hip pain in children, the child may actually feel most or all of the pain in his or her knee. Treatment is likely to involve surgery.

OBSERVATION HIP. Hip pain is common, and often isn't due to Perthe's disease or a slipped epiphysis. The other likely reason is observation hip, which simply means that there is nothing to do but observe the child get better. The cause is unknown – there may be more than one – but the pain eventually disappears as mysteriously as it came.

PAIN IN THE KNEE OR ANKLE may occasionally cause a limp (see *Pains in the joints and legs*).

LONGSTANDING LIMPING possibly since the child was very young or first started to walk, isn't normal. Rarely, it may be a sign of a deformity of the bones in the legs or a disease such as muscular dystrophy, polio or brain damage. Often there is nothing serious to find, but it should be CHECKED BY A DOCTOR.

❖　　　❖　　　❖　　　❖　　　❖

GUIDANCE
SEE YOUR DOCTOR if

❖　　you suspect that a broken bone or serious injury may be involved, OR

❖　　your child limps for no obvious reason, for more than one day, OR

❖　　there is redness or swelling of joints in the foot, ankle or knee (see *Pains in the joints and legs*), OR

❖　　there is pain in the hip or knee.

Often, the doctor will simply be able to reassure you that all seems well even though the cause is a mystery, and advise no treatment.

LUMPS, ABDOMEN

Lumps on a child's abdomen are generally harmless, although often quite worrying to parents.

AN UMBILICAL HERNIA is the most common cause. This means that the child is born with a hole in the layer of muscle and sinew that forms the front wall of the abdomen, at the **umbilicus** (navel).

The peritoneum, the tough membrane lining the inside of the child's abdomen, balloons out through this hole to form a lump under the skin. Usually this balloon of peritoneum contains a portion of the child's bowel.

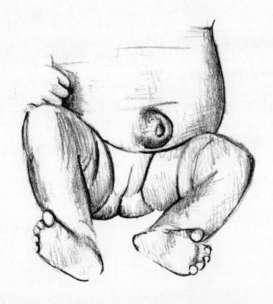

Umbilical hernias rarely cause any problems

GUIDANCE
Umbilical hernias are most common in Afro-Caribbean babies. They are harmless, and virtually never strangulate (see *Lumps, groin or testicle,* for an explanation of a strangulated hernia).

❖   ❖   ❖

The symptoms of an umbilical hernia are simply a lump right over the umbilicus which usually gets bigger and smaller, becoming big and hard when the child strains or cries, and often disappearing altogether when he or she lies quietly. Pushing the top of the lump with your finger will usually make it disappear with a gurgle.

Small hernias may just look like a swollen or prominent umbilicus, but pushing the swelling back with your finger clinches the diagnosis.

❖   ❖   ❖

Treatment is almost always unnecessary for umbilical hernias, as they disappear for good on their own, usually by the age of 18 months.

OTHER LUMPS IN THE ABDOMEN are likely to be lumps in the skin such as lipomas or sebaceous cysts (see *Lumps in the skin*).

Much more rarely, they may be lumps inside the abdomen itself, and constipation is the most likely cause. You should SEE YOUR DOCTOR if you suspect that your child has a lump in the abdomen.

LUMPS, GROIN OR TESTICLE

People are sometimes confused by the term groin. It refers to the creases in the skin where your legs join the rest of your body at the front. It doesn't include a boy's testicles or scrotum, although swellings of these are mentioned in this section.

LUMPS IN THE GROIN are usually due to swollen lymph glands, or to a hernia.

Lymph glands are present all around your body, some immediately under the skin and some deeper inside. They are part of your body's defence system against invading bugs. An infection will cause the glands to swell as they prevent the further spread of infection. Usually, this is most obvious as swelling of the glands in your neck with a cold, flu or sore throat.

SWOLLEN LYMPH GLANDS. A severe flu-like illness may cause lymph glands to swell all over a child's body, in the armpits and groin as well as in the neck. Swollen glands in just one side of the groin usually mean an infection in or around that area, such as a skin infection on one leg. A reaction to an injection in the bottom is another common cause. Swollen glands usually feel slightly soft, and may be tender; usually there will be several in the groin at once, even if one is considerably bigger than the others.

A SINGLE LUMP IN THE GROIN could be an **inguinal hernia**. This means that part of the peritoneum, the tough membrane lining the inside of the child's abdomen, is poking through a hole in the layer of muscle and sinew that forms the front wall of the abdomen. This balloon of peritoneum forms a lump under the skin; it may be empty

147

apart from some fluid, or it may contain part of the child's bowel.

In adults this type of hernia is usually the result of a strain, but in babies it is often present from birth. The swelling tends to grow bigger and smaller, becoming worse if the child strains or cries, and maybe disappearing altogether when he or she lies quietly. Sometimes both sides of the groin are affected.

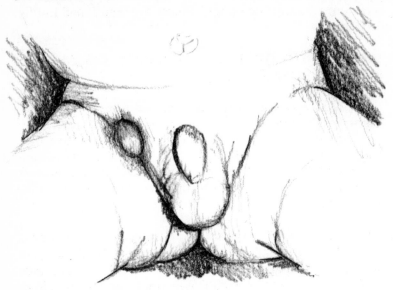

Inguinal hernias in babies need treatment by surgery

SCROTAL SWELLING. Inguinal hernias are much more common in boys than girls, and may extend into the scrotum causing a swelling here too.

This scrotal swelling may contain just fluid (a **hydrocoele**) or may also contain part of the bowel. Hydrocoeles are common immediately after birth without a hernia being present, and generally clear up on their own. Later on, a hydrocoele is likely to be a sign of a hernia. All hydrocoeles should be CHECKED BY A DOCTOR to see whether surgery is necessary.

GUIDANCE

Inguinal hernias in children won't get better on their own, and run the risk of **strangulation**. This means that a portion of bowel becomes jammed so tightly into the hernia that its blood supply is cut off. The bowel dies and serious infection and bowel blockage may result.

For this reason, the only treatment for an inguinal hernia is surgery. A hernia which becomes hard and tender for more than a couple of hours, and which you can't push back, may be strangulated and you should SEE A DOCTOR IMMEDIATELY.

A LUMP IN THE GROIN OF A BOY who doesn't have both his testicles in his scrotum, may actually be a **maldescended testicle** which hasn't moved down into the scrotum as it should.

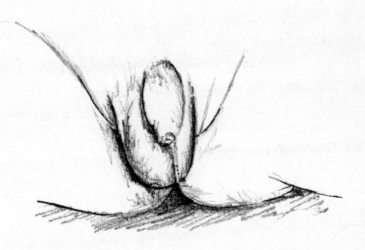

*A lump in the groin of a boy may be
a maldescended testicle*

149

GUIDANCE
SEE YOUR DOCTOR if you can't easily feel both your son's testicles in his scrotum (the doctor will also examine your son's testicles at his routine baby checks).

Often the problem is simply that the muscle which pulls the testicles right to the top of the scrotum, is over-active in small boys. This is normal; but if one or both testicles are really maldescended and don't arrive in the scrotum by the age of four or five years, then surgery to fix them in the scrotum will be necessary.

OTHER CAUSES OF LUMPS IN THE GROIN include lipomas and sebaceous cysts (see *Lumps in the skin*). These are harmless and don't usually need any treatment, although they are generally straightforward to remove by surgery if needs be.

❖　　　❖　　　❖　　　❖　　　❖

SEE YOUR DOCTOR if your child

❖　　has a single lump in one or both sides of the groin, OR

❖　　has very swollen lymph glands for no obvious reason, OR

❖　　has a swelling in his scrotum, OR

❖　　has the symptoms of a hernia.

LUMPS IN THE NECK

SEVERAL LUMPS IN THE NECK AT ONCE are common in children, and are usually due to **enlarged lymph glands** (see *Lumps, groin or testicle*). Often there will be an obvious cause such as a cold or sore throat, and glands will enlarge on both sides of the neck. They may be tender and painful, and produce a stiff neck (see *Neck, stiff or painful*).

Lymph glands feel smooth, usually slightly soft and tender, and may become quite enormous, the size of a large marble. They usually appear in the nape of the neck just below the base of the skull, in a line down the side of the neck towards the back, in another line towards the front, and at the base of the neck behind the collar bone. Although they shrink back within days or weeks, children who suffer repeated infections may have permanently enlarged glands.

Enlarged glands on just one side may be a sign of an infection in the surrounding area, such as a mouth ulcer or skin or ear infection.

GUIDANCE
Swollen glands don't mean anything in themselves; they are a sign that something, usually an infection, is going on elsewhere in the body. A generalised illness, such as flu, may cause swollen glands in the groin and armpits too.

❖　　❖　　❖

Provided that there is an obvious cause, swollen glands can generally be safely ignored, but SEE YOUR DOCTOR if they don't show any sign of shrinking after two weeks.

A SINGLE LUMP IN THE NECK may also be a lymph gland. Often, if you feel carefully, you find that other glands

151

are swollen around it, but are less obvious.

If it isn't in the right position for a lymph gland then it may be a skin lump, such as a **lipoma** or **sebaceous cyst** (see *Lumps in the skin*).

Usually, skin lumps are quite mobile and will move round as you push the skin; lymph glands are fixed deeper down and won't move as much.

GUIDANCE
Usually,the cause of a single enlarged lymph gland is an infection in the surrounding area, but rarely there may be other causes such as tuberculosis or lymphoma (a kind of cancer of the lymph glands). For this reason, **any single lump which stays in the neck for more than 10 days** should be CHECKED BY A DOCTOR.

NECK LUMPS THAT ARE PRESENT FROM BIRTH are often **congenital cysts**. These are round cysts filled with fluid or thick liquid which form due to a minor abnormality of development while the child is in the womb.

GUIDANCE
Generally they are harmless and don't mean that anything else is wrong. They should be CHECKED BY A DOCTOR though, as one rare form, called a **cystic hygroma**, may indicate problems with the system of lymph glands and the lymphatic vessels which connect them.

A large lump or swelling on one side of the neck, together with a stiff neck, may mean a sternomastoid tumour (see *Neck, stiff or painful*).

❖   ❖   ❖   ❖   ❖

Sometimes the **position of a swelling** gives a clue to its cause.

SWELLING BELOW THE EAR may be due to an **enlarged parotid gland**, one of the salivary glands that keep the mouth moist.

Mumps is the most likely cause in children; usually the child isn't too unwell, and may even have no symptoms whatsoever. Otherwise he or she may have a temperature, headache and feel generally off for a day or two before the swelling appears on one or both sides of the face. Treatment simply means keeping the child comfortable, and away from other children for seven to ten days until the swelling has gone.

GUIDANCE
Mumps is caused by a **virus infection**, and catching it once usually means that the child is immune and will never catch it again. The MMR jab, given between 12 and 15 months of age, includes protection against mumps. Sometimes, the jab itself may cause slight parotid gland swelling (see *Immunisation reactions*).

❖   ❖   ❖

A **red swollen parotid gland** may mean a blockage or infection and should be CHECKED BY A DOCTOR.

SWELLING UNDER THE JAW may be due to **enlarged submandibular glands**. Like the parotid glands, these make saliva. There is one gland on either side, under the jaw, and normally you can't feel them. **Mumps** is the most common cause of swelling, and may affect one or both sides. It may involve the parotid glands too, so that the whole side of the child's face seems puffed out.

Occasionally, in older children, a swollen submandibular gland may be due to a stone which has formed in the gland. Suspect this (and CHECK WITH YOUR DOCTOR) if the gland keeps swelling, particularly whilst eating, and then shrinking again; or if it becomes red and tender.

A SWELLING OVER THE THROAT AT THE FRONT which moves when the child swallows, may sometimes indicate an enlarged thyroid gland. This lies under the skin in front of the windpipe, just below the Adam's apple.

SEE YOUR DOCTOR if you suspect a thyroid swelling; sometimes the gland is under-active and need treatment.

❖   ❖   ❖   ❖   ❖

Although there are many other possibly causes of swellings and lumps in the neck, they are rare. SEE YOUR DOCTOR if a single lump or swelling doesn't start to go within 10 days.

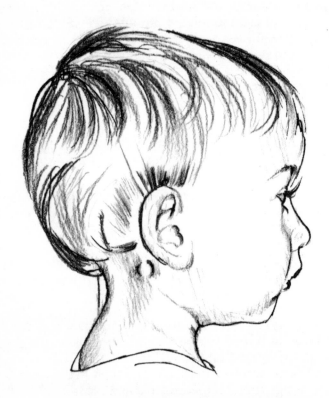

Lumps in the neck are often due to swollen lymph glands

LUMPS IN THE SKIN

Lumps in or just under the skin are usually caused by swollen lymph glands, sebaceous cysts, lipomas, and occasionally other causes.

SWOLLEN LYMPH GLANDS usually affect the neck, armpits or groin (see *Lumps, groin or testicle* and *Lumps in the neck*). Sometimes they may appear in other places, such as elbows or knees.

Although you can move them a little with your finger, they are under the skin rather than in it, and won't move with the skin when you push it.

SEBACEOUS CYSTS are sometimes called **epidermal cysts**. They form when a hair follicle, the skin pore which grows a hair, blocks and fills with thick, white, waxy material. They may appear anywhere except the palms and soles, but are most common on the scalp, face, neck and trunk. Usually they are up to one or two centimetres in diameter, but occasionally grow to several centimetres.

The cyst appears as a smooth round swelling often with a dimple or small black spot in the centre – this is the pore, the opening of the blocked follicle.

The cyst shouldn't be tender, feels tense but not hard, and moves with the skin.

GUIDANCE
Sebaceous cysts are harmless. Occasionally, they may become inflamed or infected, forming a boil (see *Boils*) and may then need surgical removal to prevent further infections. Otherwise surgery, although straightforward and effective, is really only necessary for cosmetic reasons.

LIPOMAS may look and feel similar to sebaceous cysts, although they don't have the characteristic dimple in the middle. They are lumps of fatty tissue under the skin, and may occur anywhere – particularly the neck, top of the trunk, arms and legs.

They are harmless, but can be surgically removed if they are ugly or inconvenient.

GANGLIONS may sometimes be mistaken for cysts or lipomas. They only ever occur **over tendons**, usually around the wrist or ankle. A tendon is the tough sinew that connects a muscle to a bone, and each one is surrounded by a sheath. A weakness in the sheath causes a bulge at this point, which fills with a jelly-like substance.

This bulge is a ganglion. It lies over the tendon but doesn't move when the tendon moves. It doesn't move with the skin either. Ganglions don't usually grow much bigger than about one centimetre in diameter. They are harmless and often disappear on their own; if not then they can be surgically removed, but sometimes return even then.

A RED FLESHY SWELLING APPEARING OVER A CUT OR INJURY may be a **pyogenic granuloma**. Hands and feet, sometimes lips and gums, are most commonly affected, often where a thorn or splinter has pierced the skin. The granuloma is made up of scar and inflammatory tissue; for some reason the body's healing response to the injury has gone out of control.

You should SEE YOUR DOCTOR who may arrange removal by cautery (burning the tissue away) or surgery.

HARD SWELLING AROUND A SCAR may be due to **keloid scarring**. This simply means that the body has made more hard scar tissue than normal. Some people seem particularly prone to keloid scars, which are harmless although they may look unsightly.

SEE YOUR DOCTOR, although most prefer to wait for the scar to improve with time, as treatment may make things worse. Occasionally, treatment with steroid injections or tape, and rarely surgery, will help.

A LUMP UNDER THE SKIN OF THE EYELID may be a Meibomian cyst (see *Eyes, red, sore or sticky*).

❖   ❖   ❖   ❖   ❖

SEE YOUR DOCTOR about any lump that you aren't happy about; the chances are that you will be reassured.

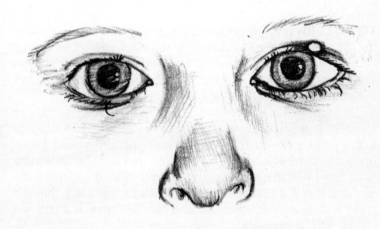

Meibomian cysts usually affect the upper eyelid

MASTURBATION

Masturbation is quite common at all ages of childhood, although it may come as a great shock to discover your own child indulging. Children who are bored, stressed or emotionally deprived, may sometimes masturbate excessively; but this is not to say that masturbation is anything but healthy and normal in other children.

TODDLERS may squeeze their legs together as they sit or lie, or may rock backwards and forwards. They may become breathless or flushed and may shout out or shriek. They may seem to be in a world of their own at the time, not noticing anything that is happening around them.

Usually it is quite easy to see what is going on, although occasionally the child may rock so violently and be so unaware of what is going on around, that it is difficult to be sure that he or she isn't having an epileptic fit. Usually the fact that there are no other features of a fit (see *Fits*), that the child isn't sleepy afterwards, and can be distracted with an effort, will confirm the diagnosis; but ASK YOUR DOCTOR if in doubt.

OLDER CHILDREN may rub or play experimentally with their genitalia. By now, they may have enough idea of the taboos surrounding sexual activity to feel ashamed or choose to do this in private.

GUIDANCE
Many of our outmoded ideas concerning masturbation date from the time of the Victorians who blamed masturbation for blindness, sterility, madness, impotence and premature old age, as well as all manner of other problems. Even the

Church used to believe that masturbation was sinful. Of course this is all nonsense; there are no harmful physical effects from masturbation, and it is quite healthy and normal even in young children.

❖　　　❖　　　❖

Treatment isn't necessary, although usually it is possible to divert your child's attention and persuade him or her to do something else if you prefer. Treating masturbation as something wrong that should be punished is likely to make you feel guilty and your child confused.

❖　　　❖　　　❖

SEE YOUR DOCTOR if you can't be sure that your child isn't really having fits.

NAPPY RASH

Any rash in a baby's nappy area is technically a nappy rash, but usually the cause is **ammoniacal dermatitis**. This means the effect of ammonia, released from stale urine, on the skin of the baby's bottom.

Ammonia inflames the skin, making it red and sore sometimes to the point where it weeps and bleeds. Creases and folds in the skin, where the ammonia can't reach, tend not to be affected.

Although regular changing and keeping the bottom dry certainly help to prevent nappy rash, some babies with sensitive skin are simply more prone to it than others. Nappy rash doesn't mean neglect, or that your care isn't adequate – it affects most babies at some time.

INFECTION is a common complication of nappy rash. Usually **thrush**, a yeast infection, is the culprit although sometimes bacteria are to blame. Thrush infection is so common that it is safest to assume that it affects any nappy rash which has been present for more than two days. Thrush infection causes the rash to become bright red; unlike ammoniacal dermatitis it affects the skin folds, and you may notice small red spots spreading up onto the baby's body.

Sometimes **thrush on the bottom** means that there is thrush elsewhere too. Check for white spots in the baby's mouth (see *Pain in the mouth and teeth*) and sore nipples if you are breast feeding.

HOME TREATMENT
Treatment of **nappy rash** usually works well, although it isn't always easy as the most effective method is simply to

leave the nappies off as much as possible – all day if you can. Expose the bare bottom to warm dry air. Wash and carefully dry the bottom whenever you can, when changing the nappy. Barrier cream, such as **zinc and castor oil**, will help protect the skin from urine and ammonia.

❖   ❖   ❖

Use one-way liners to keep the bottom dry if you are using terries, and try washing the nappies in a weak solution of one tablespoon vinegar to a gallon of water. This acts as a weak acid and neutralises ammonia on the skin. Change the nappies very frequently if you are using disposables.

❖   ❖   ❖

SEE YOUR DOCTOR if the rash hasn't started to improve in a couple of days, if it is severe, if it bleeds, or shows signs of thrush infection (see above).

DOCTOR'S TREATMENT
The doctor may suggest a mild steroid cream such as hydrocortisone to reduce soreness and inflammation, an anti-fungal cream to treat thrush, or a combination cream which contains both.

Thrush in the baby's mouth or on your nipples will need to be treated, otherwise a recurrence in the nappy area is likely.

OTHER, VERY RARE, CAUSES OF NAPPY RASH include a form of **psoriasis**, an inherited condition where skin cells are being created and lost much more quickly than normal, causing red and purple scaly patches of skin. SEE YOUR DOCTOR; this needs different treatment.

NECK, STIFF OR PAINFUL

Children often complain of a stiff or painful neck, and usually there is nothing serious going on. But neck stiffness is important because occasionally it may be a sign of meningitis (see later in this section)

A STIFF NECK IN A NEWBORN BABY isn't likely to be meningitis, although you should SEE A DOCTOR IMMEDIATELY if the child seems at all unwell (see *Ill – should your child see the doctor?*). Often the cause is a **sternomastoid tumour**. This means a swollen neck muscle, probably as a result of damage during birth. The baby won't let you turn his or her neck in one direction, and there may be a swelling on the side of the neck.

Sternomastoid tumours usually get better with a course of physiotherapy but, if they aren't treated, may occasionally lead to permanent damage to the neck muscle and a permanently twisted neck.

A PERMANENTLY STIFF OR TWISTED NECK IN OLDER CHILDREN may be the result of an **untreated sternomastoid tumour** (see above) and should be CHECKED BY A DOCTOR in case treatment with physiotherapy, injections or surgery is necessary.

A SUDDEN STIFF NECK IN OLDER CHILDREN is usually due to **muscle spasm**. Often the child wakes up with pain in the neck, usually on one side. The cause isn't known, although sitting in a draught sometimes seems to be a trigger. The child holds his or her neck to one side because of the pain, and the neck muscles on that side will be tight and tender.

With rest, heat (a hot bath or hot water bottle) and gentle

exercises, the stiffness should disappear within a week or two.

A SUDDEN STIFF NECK IN A CHILD WHO IS UNWELL, usually with an earache, a sore throat or fever, is often due to **enlarged neck glands** (see *Lumps in the neck*). Nevertheless, it must be taken seriously because of the danger of meningitis, so SEE YOUR DOCTOR.

MENINGITIS is an infection of the meninges, the membranes lining the outer surface of the brain. It generally affects children under five years of age, and is potentially dangerous, especially to babies and toddlers.

At first the child becomes generally unwell and irritable with vomiting and a temperature. Older children will develop head and neck pain with neck stiffness, but babies may simply become more and more poorly with a bulging fontanelle (the soft spot at the top of the head) and may hold their heads bent back. The child may develop fits and eventually become unconscious.

A **rash of small, flat, purplish blotches** is a sign of serious meningitis due to **meningococcus bacteria**.

In fact, many cases of meningitis are caused by **viruses**, and get better with no treatment and without any permanent damage. Meningitis caused by **bacteria** is more serious, and may cause death or permanent brain damage, if it isn't treated in time.

GUIDANCE
SEE A DOCTOR IMMEDIATELY if your child has any of the above symptoms, or if he or she has a temperature or isn't well and can't touch the chin onto the chest because of pain and stiffness in the neck.

RARER CAUSES OF A STIFF NECK include the effects of some drugs (including some anti-sickness drugs), arthritis (see *Pain in the joints and legs*), defective neck bones which haven't developed properly, and cerebral palsy which is present from birth.

OLDER CHILDREN, like adults, may develop painful stiffness and tension in the back of the neck as a result of **stress.** This may lead to a **tension headache** (see *Pains in the head*).

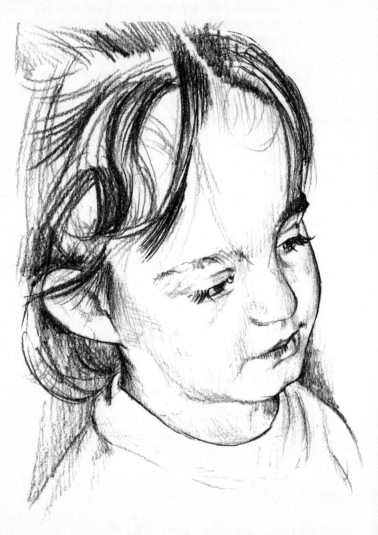

Sternomastoid tumours usually get better with a course of physiotherapy

NIGHTMARES, NIGHT TERRORS AND SLEEPWALKING

NIGHTMARES are common, and nearly all children have them at some time. Stress, anxiety or a difficult time at home or school may occasionally produce a flurry of frequent nightmares but most of the time nightmares are normal and they don't suggest any insecurity or emotional problems. Sometimes an infection such as a cold or sore throat, or a loud noise late at night, seems to start a nightmare.

Nightmares are simply bad dreams. The child will remember the dream immediately afterwards if he or she wakes, but will soon forget the details. If the child doesn't wake, then he or she may simply have a vague uneasy memory by the next morning. Sometimes a child will toss in bed and moan or even cry out during a nightmare, but unlike with night terrors or sleepwalking, the child won't sit up or get out of bed.

GUIDANCE
Usually, there is no need for treatment apart from reassurance. Leaving the bedroom door open or the light on at night may help a child who is afraid to go to bed because of nightmares.

NIGHT TERRORS are less common than nightmares, but often much more terrifying to see. Usually they start after the child has been asleep for an hour or two; the child suddenly screams and sits bolt upright in bed, maybe even getting out of bed and stumbling around the room. The child's eyes are open and he or she is staring, apparently terrified, as if being attacked by something that isn't there. He or she seems not to see you, or to hear your voice, if you are there.

GUIDANCE
Night terrors are not simply bad nightmares; in fact the two are completely different. During sleep we all pass through different levels of consciousness, known as stages or phases of sleep. **Dreams and nightmares occur in rapid eye movement (REM) sleep**, when the child's eyes move rapidly backwards and forwards under the closed eyelids as if he or she if following the action of the dream.

❖　　　❖　　　❖

Night terrors don't occur in REM sleep, and although no one is quite sure what is going on, the child certainly isn't dreaming. If you do wake your child immediately after a night terror, he or she won't remember a thing. There will be no recollection or sense of unease the next morning either.

❖　　　❖　　　❖

A night terror won't last more than a few minutes, after which the child will go soundly back to sleep again.

❖　　　❖　　　❖

Night terrors don't mean that there is any emotional or psychological problem; the child never remembers them, and within a few years they will simply stop happening.

SLEEP WALKING, like nightmares, is a common problem and usually affects children after the age of about four years. It occurs in the deep phase of sleep that starts within a couple of hours of dropping off and, as with night terrors, the child isn't dreaming at the time.

The child may get out of bed and walk round the room, maybe crawl into a wardrobe or try to perform some simple repetitive task. Occasionally, sleepwalking children will hold a conversation or do some quite complex work, although this is unusual.

GUIDANCE
Sometimes the tendency to sleepwalk seems to run in families. Usually there isn't any obvious cause, although some parents find that a large meal late at night makes their child more likely to sleepwalk.

❖   ❖   ❖

The danger of harm, for example from falling through a window or down the stairs, is really very small, although it is understandably worrying to parents.

❖   ❖   ❖

Sleepwalking doesn't point to an emotional or psychological problem and usually stops happening with time.

NOSE BLEEDS

Although nose bleeds are rare (and should be CHECKED BY A DOCTOR) in babies, they are very common in older children. Usually the cause is a knock on the nose, or an infection such as a cold, which inflames the lining of the nose and expands the delicate blood vessels inside it.

RECURRENT NOSEBLEEDS, that keep on happening, sometimes several times a week, usually mean that the blood vessels lining the inside of the nose are unusually fragile. These blood vessels group together at one point, known as **Little's area**, on the inside of the nose towards the front of the septum (the plate of gristle that separates the two nostrils). This area is prone to bleeding, and nosebleeds generally start from here.

COUGHING OR VOMITING UP BLOOD that has been swallowed, is quite common during or immediately after a nose bleed and, provided that you are sure that the blood is coming from the nose, there is no cause for concern.

Blood tends to irritate the stomach, so that any that is swallowed is quite likely to be vomited back.

MUCH RARER CAUSES OF NOSE BLEEDS include high blood pressure, and blood diseases which stop the blood from clotting normally.

A constant bloodstained discharge from just one nostril is most likely to be due to a foreign object (see *Foreign objects*).

GUIDANCE
Treatment of a nose bleed means keeping the child, and yourself, calm. Excitement or agitation is likely to make things worse and prolong the bleeding.

❖   ❖   ❖

Sit the child at a table with a large bowl in front of him or her. Tell your child to pinch very firmly just below the bony bridge of the nose, or do this yourself for a younger child. Make the child lean forward over the bowl, breathing through the mouth with the mouth constantly open, so that any blood will drip straight into the bowl.

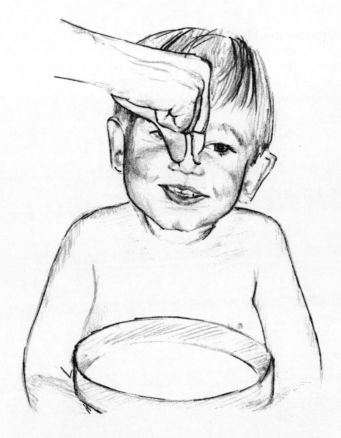

The right treatment should stop a nosebleed within 20 minutes

169

❖   ❖   ❖

This should stop a nose bleed within 20 minutes; if it doesn't THEN TAKE YOUR CHILD TO CASUALTY as, very rarely, a doctor may need to stop the bleeding by passing a gauze pack, or occasionally an inflatable rubber balloon, into the nose. **Never** try to pack the nose yourself.

❖   ❖   ❖

Treatment of recurrent nose bleeds often isn't necessary as they usually stop happening eventually. If they are a nuisance then SEE YOUR DOCTOR, who may arrange for the fragile Little's area to be **cauterised** (burned). Usually this means applying a chemical, silver nitrate, just inside the nose.

NOSE, CONSTANTLY RUNNY

A CONSTANTLY RUNNY NOSE IN BABIES is very common in the first few weeks of life. No one is quite sure of the cause; it doesn't seem to be due to allergy or infection, although it may partly be due to the small size of the passages in the baby's nose.

Occasionally it may block the baby's nose and interfere with feeding. Then, SEE YOUR DOCTOR, who may suggest sterile salt water nose drops to use before feeds.

Usually the problem gets better within a few weeks, occasionally longer.

A CONSTANTLY RUNNY NOSE IN TODDLERS AND OLDER CHILDREN is usually quite normal, too. Most children go through a so-called **catarrhal phase** some time before the age of eight years. All this means is that they are coming across so many cold and flu viruses for the first time, that they perpetually catch one cold after another.

Because they are still building up their resistance, these children can't fight their colds as effectively as adults, and the symptoms may last longer. Eventually, one cold merges into another, and besides a constantly snuffly or runny nose with thick yellow mucus, the child may have permanently huge tonsils and enlarged lymph glands in the neck (see *Lumps in the neck*).

The catarrhal phase gets better within a few years without treatment, as the child builds up resistance to different strains of cold virus.

ALLERGY is another possible cause of a constantly runny nose. The child may be allergic to pollen, house dust or other substances in the air (see *Hay fever and nose allergies*).

An allergy will often produce a constant, clear watery discharge with frequent sneezing, sometimes with red or itchy eyes and wheezing.

If your child has this combination then SEE YOUR DOCTOR.

A RUNNY NOSE JUST FROM ONE NOSTRIL usually means that there is a foreign object in the nostril (see *Foreign objects*).

PAIN IN THE ABDOMEN, LONGSTANDING

PAIN IN THE ABDOMEN THAT KEEPS COMING BACK over a period of months or even years, affects up to ten per cent of school children, and seems to be even more common between the ages of 12 and 15 years.

No physical cause can be found in about 90 per cent of cases. Often, emotion seems to be important. Sometimes there will be an obvious cause for stress, and the child may appear anxious and worried; sometimes conflicts at home or at school are to blame. At other times there may be no obvious trigger.

Some form of recurrent pain like this may be a form of **childhood migraine**, especially if other members of the family suffer migraines. The chances of a child who has suffered bouts of abdominal pain developing true migraine headaches in later life, are considerably greater than normal.

This **'non-organic' pain** without a physical cause often appears around the child's umbilicus as a constant dull ache. Vomiting and headaches are common during an attack; the child may turn pale and may go to sleep afterwards. The pain may occur day or night, but doesn't usually wake the child up. Often it crops up several times a week for weeks on end, then disappears altogether for some months before appearing again.

HOME TREATMENT
Treatment for this kind of pain really just means keeping your child comfortable while waiting for the pains to stop on their own after a few years.

❖   ❖   ❖

Your child is in real pain and isn't simply seeking attention or time off school, even though there is no physical cause.

❖   ❖   ❖

Paracetamol (see dosage, page 11) and a hot bath or hot water bottle may help.

OTHER CAUSES OF RECURRENT ABDOMINAL PAIN are less common.

Occasionally, **repeated urine infections** can cause longstanding pain in the back or low in the abdomen. SEE YOUR DOCTOR, who may check a sample of urine to rule this out.

Constipation probably isn't as common a cause of abdominal pains as people often think. Most children with constipation don't have pain, although actually opening their bowels may hurt. Sometimes a feeling of fullness and discomfort low in the abdomen, which gets better after opening the bowels, may be due to constipation.

Severe constipation should always be CHECKED BY YOUR DOCTOR (see *Constipation*).

Black Afro-Caribbean children with repeated bouts of pain may be suffering from **sickle cell disease** (see *Pain in the abdomen, sudden*).

A grumbling appendix used to be a common diagnosis. Then, doctors thought that repeated minor infections of the appendix could cause recurring bouts of pain, until full-blown appendicitis eventually followed after months or years (see **Appendicitis** in *Pain in the abdomen, sudden*). Nowadays, most doctors don't believe that there is any such condition as a grumbling appendix.

❖   ❖   ❖   ❖   ❖

GUIDANCE
SEE YOUR DOCTOR with a child with recurrent abdominal pain if

❖   the pain doesn't fit the description of 'non-organic' pain given above, OR

❖   the pain isn't in the centre of the abdomen (as a general rule the further the pain is from the middle, the more likely there is to be a physical cause), OR

❖   other symptoms, such as diarrhoea, constipation or vomiting, are severe, OR

❖   there are any symptoms involving the urine (see *Urine symptoms*), OR

❖   your child's rate of growth and weight gain is less than it should be (this is a good overall indicator of the state of health and whether anything serious could be going on), OR

❖   your child is ill (see *Ill – should your child see the doctor?*).

PAIN IN THE ABDOMEN, SUDDEN

SUDDEN PAIN IN THE ABDOMEN is common at all ages. There are dozens of possible causes, some of which are potentially serious and, as a general rule, **any child with an unexplained pain lasting more than three hours, or who is ill** (see *Ill - should your child see a doctor?*), **should** SEE A DOCTOR.

Sometimes it is possible to recognise one of the common or important causes described below.

PAIN IN THE ABDOMEN IN BABIES may be due to **colic** (see *Colic*), or more rarely **intussusception** (see *Blood in the stools*).

REPEATED COUGHING OR VOMITING often causes pain in the abdomen due to pulled or strained muscles. The muscles down the front of the child's abdomen may be slightly tender, but there shouldn't be any tenderness deeper inside.

A STITCH is a common cause of pain in the upper part of the abdomen, or the lower part of the chest (see *Pain in the chest*).

STOMACH BUGS CAUSING DIARRHOEA AND VOMITING may cause **colicky pains,** usually in the middle or left side of the abdomen, which are severe for a minute or two at a time, before easing off. The child may be a little uncomfortable if you press the abdomen but shouldn't be really tender and won't object to walking or rolling into a ball (see **Appendicitis**, which follows).

Usually, the diarrhoea and vomiting is quite severe, unlike the one or two bouts which may occur with appendicitis.

APPENDICITIS usually occurs in children over the age of two years. It means that the appendix, a small loop of bowel in the lower right-hand corner of the abdomen, is inflamed and infected. However, the child may not always feel the pain exactly over the appendix.

Sometimes the pain starts in the centre of the abdomen around the umbilicus, often eventually spreading to the lower right corner within a few hours. Walking or moving makes the pain worse, and the child may not be able to curl up into a ball because of pain.

Almost always the child will lose his or her appetite, feel sick, and may vomit once or twice. He or she is likely to have a slight temperature and a coated tongue. There may be constipation, or sometimes slight diarrhoea.

The most reliable sign of appendicitis is tenderness in the lower right corner of the abdomen.

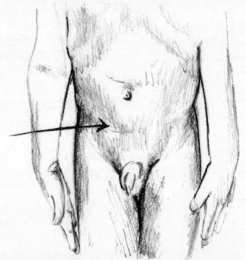

The most reliable sign of appendicitis is tenderness in the lower right corner of the abdomen

DOCTOR'S TREATMENT
SEE YOUR DOCTOR AT ONCE if you have any suspicion
of appendicitis, since the only treatment is by operation to
remove the appendix (**appendicectomy**). Without
treatment, an inflamed appendix may burst, releasing
infection into the abdominal cavity (**peritonitis**) with the
possibility of serious illness.

COLDS AND SORE THROATS often cause abdominal
pain in toddlers and young children due to **mesenteric
adenitis**. This means that lymph glands inside the child's
abdomen become swollen, painful and tender as a result of
infection, in just the same way as glands in other places (see
Lumps in the neck). This causes pain which can be very
difficult to tell apart from appendicitis.

A young child with abdominal pain and a fever, sore throat
and enlarged glands in the neck, armpits and groin,
probably has mesenteric adenitis. But the possible
consequences of missing appendicitis are so severe that you
should SEE YOUR DOCTOR to check the diagnosis.

**PAIN IN THE SIDE OF THE ABDOMEN TOWARDS
THE BACK** may be due to a kidney infection. Usually, the
child will have a fever with vomiting, and older children
may pass urine more frequently and complain of pain when
they do. Kidney stones, although rare in children, may
produce similar symptoms. SEE YOUR DOCTOR if you
suspect a urine or kidney infection (see *Urine symptoms*).

CHEST INFECTIONS may cause pain which the child feels
in the upper part of the abdomen, usually on one side or the
other.

**ABDOMINAL PAIN WITH A SWELLING IN THE
GROIN OR TESTICLE** may be due to a **strangulated
hernia** (see *Lumps, groin or testicle*) or a **twisted testicle**
(see *Pain in the testicle*) and should be CHECKED BY A
DOCTOR IMMEDIATELY.

ABDOMINAL PAIN WITH A YELLOW SKIN COLOUR is most likely to mean **infectious hepatitis** (see *Jaundice*).

ABDOMINAL PAIN IN BLACK AFRO-CARIBBEAN CHILDREN may be caused by **sickle cell disease**. This means that red blood cells are deformed and may suddenly block the blood supply to one or more areas of the body, causing great pain.

SEE YOUR DOCTOR; a single blood test will check whether your child has sickle cell disease.

EATING SOMETHING THAT HE OR SHE SHOULDN'T can cause pains in a child's abdomen, although probably not as often as people sometimes think. Sometimes you know that your child always reacts to large amounts of fruit or other food in this way, but don't be tempted to put abdominal pain down to diet unless you are sure that there is no other cause. CHECK WITH YOUR DOCTOR if in doubt.

❖　　❖　　❖　　❖　　❖

This section can give only a few pointers to the diagnosis. Unless you are sure of the cause of a sudden abdominal pain which has lasted for more than three hours, or if your child is ill (see *Ill – should your child see the doctor?*), then SEE A DOCTOR.

PAIN IN THE CHEST

Severe or long-lasting chest pain isn't very common in children, although they may quite normally experience brief flitting pains across the chest from time to time, particularly if they are ill for any other reason.

A STITCH is probably the most common cause of pain in the lower part of the chest, usually at the front on just one side. Strenuous exercise, or sometimes a meal, may trigger it, and the pain should get better after a few minutes rest.

No one is sure just what causes stitches, although the pain may be due to strain on the ligaments attaching the diaphragm – the sheet of muscle separating the chest from the abdomen – to the ribs.

STRESS OR ANXIETY may cause pains almost anywhere, including the chest. Usually the pain moves around, and is difficult to pin down.

CHEST PAIN WHICH IS WORSE ON BREATHING AND COUGHING is known as **pleuritic pain**. It should be taken seriously because it may be a sign of a problem with the lungs or the pleura, the membrane between the lungs and the rib-cage.

Pleuritic pain in children may mean **pneumonia**, particularly if there are other signs such as a cough and temperature (see *Cough and cold*). SEE YOUR DOCTOR if your child has pleuritic pain.

CHEST PAIN WHICH IS WORSE ON MOVING is more likely to be due to **an injury**, even though there may be little or no bruising or signs of damage. Usually, the child will be tender over the affected area, too. As with pleuritic pain, this pain will be affected by coughing or deep breaths, but moving or pressing the area will make it worse.

A pain restricted to **one part of the rib-cage** which is also very tender, may be due to a **broken rib**, especially if it was the result of a fairly violent injury. Suspect this if pressing on your child's breast bone causes pain in the affected area.

Broken ribs heal on their own with no treatment, although this may take several weeks. Even so, you should SEE YOUR DOCTOR if you suspect a broken rib, to confirm the diagnosis and to check that the lungs haven't been damaged.

BURNING PAIN BEHIND THE BREAST BONE may be **heartburn**, a burning sensation – usually after food – which is well known to many adults. It is caused by acid in the stomach leaking into the **oesophagus** (gullet) and is quite common in children, too. Some children seem particularly prone to it.

Avoiding foods which you know trigger the symptoms, sitting upright during and after meals, and taking antacid mixtures from the chemist, will usually control the problem. If not, SEE YOUR DOCTOR; more powerful drugs from him or her will help.

SHARP PAINS BEHIND THE BREAST BONE with a cold or sore throat may be due to **tracheitis**. This means an inflamed windpipe, caused by the same virus that is responsible for the sore throat. Often the child will have a dry cough too. Tracheitis will get better within a few days. Paracetamol (see dosage, page 11) and breathing steam (see *Colds*) will help to control the pain.

CHEST PAIN AFTER A FEW DAYS' COUGH is common, and usually means that your child has simply sprained one of the muscles between his or her ribs through coughing. Moving and pressing on the affected area may be painful too.

The pain will disappear soon after the cough gets better, but if you have any suspicion that the pain may really be **pleuritic** (see above) then SEE YOUR DOCTOR.

PAIN OR DISCHARGE IN THE EAR

Earache is common in children of all ages, and some children seem more prone to it than others.

GOING OUT IN THE COLD affects some children, although the earache should get better within a few minutes, once the child reaches warmth.

GUIDANCE
Hats or ear muffs will help to prevent the problem, but don't be tempted to put cotton wool or anything else into your child's ear.

❖   ❖   ❖

Putting anything into your child's ear is always **best avoided**. It doesn't do a very good job of clearing wax or anything else from the ear, and may trigger **otitis externa** (see below) or damage the ear drum. Cotton wool in the ear may break up and be difficult to remove. Cotton wool-tipped ear buds may actually make ear wax worse.

AN EAR INFECTION is a common cause of earache, particularly up to the age of eight years. Usually there is an infection of the middle ear, the part behind the ear drum, and this is known as **otitis media**. The child may have a cold for a few days beforehand; once the ear infection appears the child will probably develop a temperature, and may vomit. If he or she is old enough, the child will complain of pain in the ear, and may become deaf on that side. Babies and younger children may simply become hot, screaming and miserable.

During the infection the middle ear fills with fluid and pus, and sometimes this causes so much pressure that the ear drum bursts. This leaves a hole in the ear drum – a **perforation** – and causes a discharge as the fluid leaks out. Often the child's pain will suddenly disappear at the same time, as the perforation releases the painful pressure on the ear drum.

GUIDANCE
You should SEE YOUR DOCTOR. **Treatment of otitis media** is usually with a course of antibiotics, although doctors' opinion is divided. Some point out that these infections seem to get better just as reliably without treatment, although it does seem that antibiotics provide a cure more quickly. Paracetamol helps pain and fever (see dosage, page 11).

❖   ❖   ❖

Occasionally fluid which has built up inside the ear doesn't drain away after the infection has cleared; antibiotic treatment may help to prevent this, but not always. For this reason you should TAKE YOUR CHILD TO THE DOCTOR six to eight weeks after a bout of otitis media, to check that the fluid has cleared. Although perforations usually heal on their own, your doctor may want to check the ear drum more frequently if a perforation has occurred. Fluid which doesn't drain can cause glue ear and deafness (see *Hearing problems*).

AN INFECTION IN THE EAR CANAL, the short tube connecting the ear drum to the outside, is less common than a middle ear infection but can be very painful. It is known as **otitis externa**, and isn't always due to an infection – sometimes the ear canal is simply inflamed by a form of dermatitis. The child will have earache, but without the fever or other symptoms that middle ear infections can cause. Often there will also be a discharge from the affected ear. You should SEE YOUR DOCTOR.

GUIDANCE
Some children seem particularly prone to otitis externa and may suffer from it repeatedly. Sometimes you can spot a trigger, such as swimming pool or bath water entering the ear.

❖   ❖   ❖

Ear drops from your doctor should provide a cure, although sometimes **aural toilet** – carefully picking out dead skin, pus and other debris from the ear canal – is necessary, usually in hospital.

❖   ❖   ❖

Although painful and a nuisance, otitis externa doesn't lead to the hearing problems that middle ear infections can cause.

A SORE THROAT OR TOOTHACHE is a surprisingly common cause of earache. The ear is particularly prone to **referred pain**; that is, the child actually feels the pain in one place although the pain itself is occurring in a different place. A sore throat or toothache may cause pain in the ear as well as, or even instead of, in the throat or teeth.

Referred earache tends to vary rather than be constant, but it may be impossible to be sure that there isn't a cause in the ear without CHECKING WITH YOUR DOCTOR.

A BOIL ON THE EAR can be very painful (see *Boils*) and it is usually obvious, although may be difficult to spot if it lies right inside the ear canal.

A FOREIGN OBJECT IN THE EAR may cause pain, usually with a discharge too (see *Foreign objects*).

EAR WAX, contrary to what many people think, very rarely causes pain. In fact it doesn't often cause any problems at all in children, and is more likely to cause deafness if anything. Rarely, a hard lump of wax which becomes impacted, or stuck, in the ear canal may cause pain.

AN INJURY TO THE EAR may cause pain, usually from bruising around the outside of the ear. A blow directly on to the ear, particularly with a flat object such as the palm of a hand, carries the risk of damage to the eardrum.

SEE YOUR DOCTOR if your child has had this kind of blow, or complains of ringing in the ear or hearing that isn't normal for more than five minutes after the injury.

EARACHE WITH DISCHARGE may mean a middle ear infection with a perforation (see above), otitis externa (see above), or a foreign object in the ear (see *Foreign objects*).

AN EAR DISCHARGE WITHOUT PAIN could also be due to any of those reasons just mentioned, but sometimes there isn't really a discharge at all. What you are seeing are runny, semi-liquid, brown or dark yellow fragments of ear wax that are escaping from the ear in the normal way. This tends to happen constantly and is normal, although you should CHECK WITH YOUR DOCTOR if you have any suspicion of a true discharge.

❖   ❖   ❖   ❖   ❖

As a general rule, SEE YOUR DOCTOR if your child has an ear discharge, or an earache that lasts for more than 20 minutes.

PAIN IN THE HEAD

Headaches are surprisingly common in children. Around one in five junior school children, and as many as 85 per cent of secondary school children, experience headaches from time to time. Some of these children have quite regular or recurrent headaches which may interfere with schooling.

A SUDDEN HEADACHE, in a child who isn't normally prone to them, usually appears as part of a cold, sore throat, flu or other bug. Sometimes a headache is the first sign that the infection is on its way. This is quite normal and can simply be treated with paracetamol (see dosage, page 11), provided that the child isn't ill (see *Ill – should your child see the doctor?*) and doesn't have any signs of meningitis (see *Neck, stiff or painful*).

Sometimes an injury is the cause of a sudden headache (see *Head injuries*). Earache or toothache can sometimes cause headache through referred pain (explained in *Pain or discharge in the ear*).

HEADACHES THAT KEEP RETURNING are more common, and often more of a problem. **Migraine** is one cause, and sometimes gives different symptoms in children and adults – although migraine is more likely in a child if one or both parents, or other members of the family, are affected.

Migraine headaches generally affect just one side of the head, and may cause vomiting with flashes or blind spots before the eyes.

Hunger and some foods, particularly cheese, chocolate and beef extract, may trigger them; sometimes stress or tiredness will set them off.

GUIDANCE
Treatment of migraine may simply involve rest and paracetamol (see dosage, page 11) at the start of an attack, and avoiding trigger foods and situations.

❖   ❖   ❖

SEE YOUR DOCTOR since other drugs he or she may prescribe, taken either regularly to prevent attacks or just when an attack starts, are usually very effective.

EYE STRAIN, contrary to what many people believe, doesn't often cause headaches. If reading seems to trigger headaches, then it is WORTH SEEING AN OPTICIAN to have your child's eyesight checked, but more often than not, glasses don't provide a cure.

BRAIN TUMOURS obviously worry parents when a child has recurrent headaches, although they are actually an extremely rare and unlikely cause – they affect about 0.005 per cent of all children.

GUIDANCE
Signs that should be CHECKED BY A DOCTOR include:

❖   headaches that don't get better with paracetamol, OR

❖   headaches that are steadily getting worse or wake the child up at night, OR

❖   continuous vomiting, OR

❖   blurred vision, double vision or crossed eyes, OR

❖   recurrent headaches in a child under five years old.

MOST RECURRENT HEADACHES aren't due to any of the above causes, and there is simply no physical explanation. Often stress or tension seems to be the cause.

Usually the headache is on both sides or all over the head, and the child may describe it as a heavy or full sensation.

Older children may experience the adult type of **tension headache**, with pain in the back of the neck or behind the eyes spreading over the head to the top.

Tension headache is actually caused by tension in the muscles in the child's neck and forehead. Sometimes there will be an obvious trigger, such as the start of a school week or the stress of exams, although these headaches may well appear out of the blue.

HOME TREATMENT
Treatment means reassuring the child and trying to help with the cause of any stress or anxiety.

❖   ❖   ❖

Paracetamol (see dosage, page 11) helps the pain, but give it as soon as the headache starts; it may not work if you leave it until the headache is well established.

❖   ❖   ❖   ❖   ❖

SEE YOUR DOCTOR if your child has recurrent headaches with any of the symptoms listed in **Brain tumours**, above; if there are symptoms of **migraine**; or if you are worried.

PAIN IN THE JOINTS AND LEGS

Leg pains are common in children, and usually don't suggest any serious problem, although there are one or two conditions to watch out for.

A SUDDEN PAIN IN ONE JOINT is usually due to an accident or injury (see *Cuts, scrapes and bruises*). An unexplained painful and swollen joint should be CHECKED BY A DOCTOR.

SUDDEN SEVERE LEG PAIN IN BLACK AFRO-CARIBBEAN CHILDREN may be due to a **sickle cell crisis** (see *Pain in the abdomen, sudden*).

A RED SWOLLEN JOINT should always be CHECKED BY A DOCTOR STRAIGHT AWAY, due to the possibility of an infection in the joint (**septic arthritis**) or a form of rheumatoid arthritis (**Still's disease,** or **juvenile rheumatoid arthritis**).

Septic arthritis can cause permanent joint damage if it isn't treated. Still's disease can damage the eyes if it isn't spotted in time.

JOINT PAINS WITH STIFFNESS particularly in the morning, or **JOINT PAINS IN A CHILD WHO IS GENERALLY UNWELL** should be taken seriously. SEE YOUR DOCTOR as they might suggest Still's disease or, rarely, leukaemia.

JOINT PAINS ALL OVER IN A CHILD WITH FLU or some other bug are very common, and are simply part of the flu-like reaction. Paracetamol should help (see dosage, page 11) and the pains will get better within a few days.

If any joints are red, swollen or stiff then SEE YOUR DOCTOR.

PAINS IN THE HIPS may have several causes (see *Limping*).

PAINS IN THE KNEE may actually be caused by a **hip problem** (see *Limping*).

In older children and adolescents, **Osgood Schlatter's disease** is common. This causes sharp pain over the front of the lower part of the knee, where the tough tendon from the kneecap joins the tibia (lower leg bone). This area might be tender to the touch. The cause is unknown although the condition is common in sporty or athletic children and it may simply be the result of damage to the leg bone where the tendon joins it.

GUIDANCE
Treatment is usually completely unnecessary as Osgood Schlatter's disease clears on its own, usually in a matter of months.

PAINS IN THE ELBOW are common in toddlers. Usually the cause is a **pulled elbow**, and although there isn't very much pain, the child won't use the arm or bend the elbow.

What has happened is that the top of the radius, one of the bones in the arm, has pulled partly through the tough ring of cartilage (gristle) that surrounds it and holds it in place.

Usually this is the result of a yank on the elbow, and it is the reason why small children shouldn't be lifted up violently by their hands.

GUIDANCE
Treatment for a **pulled elbow** is simply a matter of pushing it back into place. You can try this yourself, **provided** that there is no sign of a broken bone or other damage (see *Cuts, scrapes and bruises*).

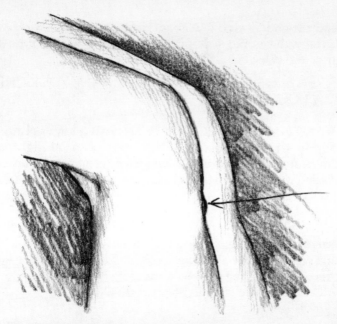

Osgood Schlatter's disease causes sharp pain where the tendon from the kneecap joins the lower leg bone

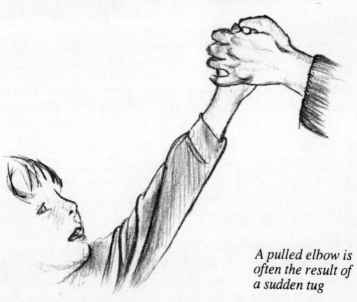

A pulled elbow is often the result of a sudden tug

Bend the child's elbow to about ninety degrees, push gently on the wrist while supporting the elbow with your other hand, and twist the wrist outwards as you push.

Try this **once only**; if it doesn't work, TAKE YOUR CHILD TO A DOCTOR.

CRAMPS IN THE LEGS are common at all ages although nobody knows the cause. They often occur at night, and sometimes after exercise. Besides excruciating pain, the affected muscle – usually in the calves – goes tight and hard into spasm.

GUIDANCE
Sometimes keeping your child's legs warmer, or cooler, in bed seems to help; the weight of bedclothes seems to trigger cramp in some people and a cage of some sort to keep the bedclothes off the feet might be worth a try.

❖   ❖   ❖

Some doctors use quinine to treat cramps, and you can try a dose of tonic water which contains quinine.

❖   ❖   ❖

When your child does get cramp, there isn't much you can do apart from rubbing and gently stretching the affected muscle for a few minutes until it clears.

❖   ❖   ❖

Cramp isn't generally a sign of anything more serious, but SEE YOUR DOCTOR if your child is getting recurrent cramps day and night, to rule out rare causes such as a deficiency of calcium or Vitamin D.

GROWING PAINS are probably the commonest cause of pains in the legs. Many doctors nowadays don't use the term growing pains, as normal growth doesn't hurt and has nothing to do with the cause of these pains. However, as there isn't really anything better to call them, the term will stick for the time being.

The pains are a bit of a mystery. They tend to affect the areas where tendons (sinews that connect muscles to bones) join the bones, and may simply be due to strain on these tendons during everyday activity. They usually affect the child's legs, and tend to be sharp flitting pains that come and go quite quickly. They are often worse at night.

Although annoying, they aren't usually very severe, and won't cause the child great pain or stop him or her doing what he or she wants to. Exercise and exertion doesn't seem to affect the pains.

GUIDANCE
Whatever they are, growing pains are harmless and can be treated with reassurance, and paracetamol (see dosage, page 11) if necessary.

❖   ❖   ❖

They may come and go for some time, months or even years, but will always disappear in the end.

PAIN IN THE MOUTH AND TEETH

TOOTHACHE isn't very common in children, but is likely to mean **disease of the tooth or gum** if it does occur.

Sometimes a child with pain in the ear or jaw will actually feel the pain in a tooth. This is **referred pain** (see *Pain or discharge in the ear*) and is common in the face and mouth. Usually a referred toothache will be more vague and difficult to pin-point than a genuine tooth pain.

Although they don't very often develop toothache, children are, unfortunately, very prone to the beginnings of **tooth decay**, which will lead to problems in later life. As many as 75 per cent of five-year-olds, and 95 per cent of 15-year-olds, have decay in at least one tooth. Fortunately, this does seem to be improving, but we still eat more sweets in this country than anywhere else in the world.

GUIDANCE
Prevention of tooth decay means regular brushing from the day the first tooth appears and avoiding too many sweets and sugary foods.

❖   ❖   ❖

Children who are too young for a fluoride toothpaste, should have extra fluoride drops if the local water supply doesn't contain much fluoride – ASK YOUR WATER COMPANY OR HEALTH VISITOR.

❖   ❖   ❖

Toothache should be CHECKED BY A DENTIST.

A SORE MOUTH IN BABIES often means **thrush**, a yeast infection. The baby may seem fine until he or she tries to feed, then will bring the mouth off the bottle or nipple after a few sucks and cry. The mouth is likely to be red inside, with white fluffy spots on the tongue and inside the cheeks.

The spots may look like milk curds, which are normal in a baby's mouth for some time after a feed. To tell the difference, try to gently scrape the spots off with the blunt end of a spoon. Milk curds will scrape off, but thrush spots will stay behind.

A baby with thrush in the mouth may well have thrush at the other end too, causing a nappy rash (see *Nappy rash*). If you are breast-feeding, your nipples may also be infected, and feel sore.

GUIDANCE
Treatment means being absolutely meticulous about sterilising teats and bottles, and treating your nipples with an anti-fungal cream such as nystatin or clotrimazole from the chemist.

❖ ❖ ❖

For your baby's mouth, use miconazole gel from the chemist which you can smear on to the inside of the mouth from the tip of your finger. Drops and lozenges are available too.

A SORE MOUTH IN OLDER CHILDREN is usually caused by **herpetic stomatitis**. This is an infection with the herpes virus, which is also responsible for cold sores.

Besides a sore mouth, children with herpetic stomatitis may be generally quite ill and have a fever and tiredness. The mouth can be so sore that the child refuses even to drink, and dribbles because of being unable even to swallow his or her own saliva. The lips, tongue, gums and inside of the mouth are covered with small blisters and ulcers. Glands in the neck may be very swollen.

GUIDANCE
Although this is a miserable condition and there is no treatment, it does get better on its own. The severe pain lasts for a few days, and the ulcers finally disappear after about ten days.

❖   ❖   ❖

Try to get your child to drink as much as you possibly can; the only danger is of dehydration because the child simply won't drink (see **Dehydration** in *Vomiting*).

❖   ❖   ❖

Clean the child's teeth as best you can; although the temptation is to leave well alone while everything is so sore, this increases the risk of secondary infections with thrush or bacteria on top of the herpes infection.

❖   ❖   ❖

SEE YOUR DOCTOR if your child has **stomatitis** and isn't drinking or there are signs of **dehydration** (see *Vomiting*). In severe cases, hospital admission, so that fluids can be dripped intravenously into a vein, is necessary.

OTHER VIRUSES may occasionally cause stomatitis similar to herpetic stomatitis. One, the **coxsackie virus**, may cause blisters on the hands and feet too (**hand, foot and mouth disease**).

A MOUTH ULCER, sometimes a crop of two or more ulcers at once, is a more common cause of mouth pain in older children. Unlike herpetic stomatitis there are only one or two ulcers, and the child is generally well, although there may be some swelling of the glands in the neck. The ulcer appears as a pale white or yellow rim around a grey centre, and is tender and painful.

Sometimes ulcers appear out of the blue, although often an injury to the inside of the child's mouth – the result of a sharp piece of food, biting the cheek or putting something hard into the mouth – scratches the lining of the mouth and sets up an ulcer.

Mouth ulcers like this are known as **aphthous ulcers**, and they get better on their own after about five days.

GUIDANCE
Although the ulcer is tender, don't be tempted to forget about tooth cleaning. This could lead to the danger of secondary infections on top of the ulcer.

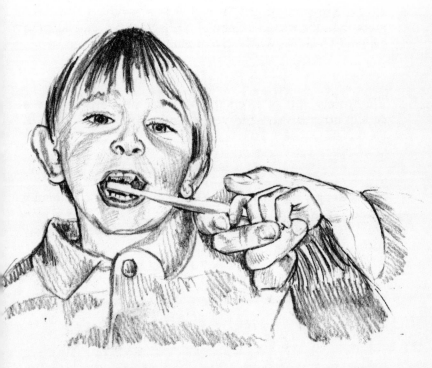

Regular teeth cleaning, even with a painful mouth, helps prevent secondary infections

❖   ❖   ❖

Anaesthetic gel or paste from the chemist might help to soothe the pain.

❖   ❖   ❖

If your child is in a great deal of pain, ASK YOUR DOCTOR about **steroid paste or tablets** to apply to the ulcer to speed its healing.

❖   ❖   ❖

Everyone has mouth ulcers from time to time; children who are generally run down through stress or illness may have more than their share. Regular tooth cleaning, and keeping generally healthy, will help to prevent them.

❖   ❖   ❖

Very rarely, lots of ulcers that keep coming back may be a sign of other disease and you should CHECK WITH YOUR DOCTOR.

❖   ❖   ❖   ❖   ❖

Some drugs, especially some antibiotics, may occasionally cause a sore mouth. CHECK WITH YOUR DOCTOR if your child develops a sore mouth, gums or lips while taking any form of medication.

PAIN IN THE TESTICLES

A boy's testicles are very sensitive and pain is usually the result of an injury or blow. Any pain which can't be explained in this way, or where the testicle is swollen, should be CHECKED AT ONCE BY A DOCTOR.

AN INJURY TO THE TESTICLE usually happens after a fight, an accident during playing or, in older boys, after rough sports. Usually the agony settles within a few minutes.

However, a more severe blow may cause bleeding inside the testicle itself which becomes swollen and very painful for several days.

An even more severe injury may split the tough coat around the outside of the testicle, causing bleeding into the scrotum which may become hugely swollen and bruised.

GUIDANCE
Usually, there is no treatment apart from painkillers such as paracetamol (see dosage, page 11), rest and warm flannels. Ice may help immediately after the injury, but don't apply it for more than a few minutes at a time.

❖   ❖   ❖

If the pain is severe, lasts longer than six hours, or there is obvious swelling or bruising, then SEE YOUR DOCTOR. Although he or she probably won't recommend any different treatment other than stronger painkillers, occasionally an operation to remove the blood and relieve the pressure on the testicle is necessary.

❖   ❖   ❖

Although painful, injuries to the testicles generally heal without permanent damage or danger to the boy's fertility in future.

PAIN IN THE TESTICLE WITHOUT INJURY should always be taken seriously, because of the risk of torsion of the testis.

Torsion of the testis means that the testicle has twisted round inside the scrotum. Normally a boy's testicles are firmly attached to the back of the scrotum making it impossible for them to twist in this way. But in some boys the testicles aren't firmly fixed, and may suddenly twist around. The danger is that this will also twist the blood vessels leading to the testicle, shutting off the blood supply with the risk of permanent damage or even the loss of the testicle.

Usually the twist causes sudden and severe pain in the testicle, often with vomiting. Sometimes the boy feels pain in the lower part of his abdomen too. The testicle will be tender and may be pulled right up to the top of the scrotum, and the testicle and scrotum gradually swell over the next few hours.

DOCTOR'S TREATMENT
You should SEE YOUR DOCTOR or GO TO CASUALTY IMMEDIATELY if you suspect **torsion of the testis**.

Treatment is by emergency surgery, to untwist the testicle and fix it properly in place. A delay could mean that the testicle is permanently damaged and needs to be removed.

INFECTIONS OF THE TESTICLE may also cause pain and, although they are usually less serious than torsion, you should CHECK WITH YOUR DOCTOR to be sure of the diagnosis.

Epididymitis is an infection of the epididymis, the collection of tubes running along the top of the testicle which carry sperm. It usually affects men, although older boys may occasionally suffer from it. The testicle and one side of the scrotum becomes swollen, tender, red and hot.

The cause is an infection with bacteria, and a course of antibiotics usually provides a cure.

MUMPS may cause swelling and pain in the testicles, and may, rarely, damage the boy's fertility in the future, although it is very uncommon for it to affect the testicles at all before puberty.

SWELLING OF THE TESTICLE with or without pain, may be caused by a **hernia** or **hydrocoele** (see *Lumps, groin or testicle*).

A MISSING TESTICLE shouldn't generally be a cause of pain, but should be CHECKED BY A DOCTOR (see *Lumps, groin or testicle*, for a **maldescended testicle**).

A SUDDEN, STEADY PAIN IN THE TESTICLE should always be CHECKED BY A DOCTOR because of the risk of **torsion of the testis**.

PALENESS

A pale complexion doesn't usually suggest any disease or problem, but is more likely simply to be the colouring that the child has been born with.

SUDDEN PALENESS is often a sign of a cold, flu or other infection. There may be bouts of fever mixed with bouts of shivering.

Since body heat is lost from blood in the skin, the child's body shuts off some of the blood supply to the skin in order to conserve heat and raise his or her body temperature. At other times the skin may become red and flushed as the body tries to get rid of excess heat.

AN EMOTIONAL UPSET OR SUDDEN SHOCK may cause paleness in older children and adolescents, sometimes as the first sign of a faint (see *Fainting*).

SEVERE PAIN may cause paleness, as the heart beats more slowly and the blood pressure drops.

SUDDEN PALENESS IN BABIES may be due to pain from **intussusception** (see *Pain in the abdomen, sudden*) or **colic** (see *Crying babies*).

SHOCK is an important cause of sudden paleness. This is the **medical use of the term shock**; the child has a fast pulse, rapid breathing, is pale, cold and sweaty or clammy.

Shock is a sign that the child's circulation is failing. It may be due to the sudden loss of a large amount of blood, or the loss of other fluid such as with severe vomiting or diarrhoea. Severe allergy or infection may place such a strain that the the child's heart isn't able to cope, and he or she develops shock. Other causes, such as heart disease, are much less common.

Fortunately shock is very rare, but it is a **medical emergency**. DIAL 999 AND GET MEDICAL HELP IMMEDIATELY.

PALENESS OVER A LONG PERIOD OF TIME is likely simply to be the child's natural complexion. Occasionally, **anaemia** is to blame.

ANAEMIA means that the child doesn't have enough red blood cells. These are cells which carry oxygen in the blood to all the body's tissues, and which give blood its deep red colour. Paleness is one sign of anaemia but, unfortunately, it isn't always a very reliable one as so many children simply have naturally pale skin.

Signs of anaemia that are more reliable include paleness of the tongue, of the inside of the mouth and of the red area that is exposed when you pull down the child's lower eyelid. The fingertips under the nails may be pale too. With severe anaemia the child may be tired (see *Tiredness*), and become short of breath with a racing pulse after slight exercise. If the anaemia continues, it may slow the child's growth.

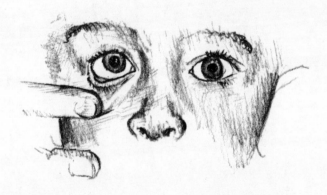

Look for paleness of the red area that is exposed when you pull down the child's lower eyelid

203

There are dozens of possible **causes of anaemia**. Loss of blood, possibly from an injury, nosebleeds or invisible bleeding into the bowel, may be responsible. Sometimes the child's diet doesn't contain enough iron or vitamins; this is a risk in babies who are breast-fed for many months without vitamin supplements. Infections, some drugs, and blood disorders such as sickle cell disease (see *Pain in the abdomen, sudden*) or leukaemia, may also be to blame.

DOCTOR'S TREATMENT
Treatment of **anaemia** means first confirming the diagnosis and finding the cause. SEE YOUR DOCTOR who will probably arrange a blood test to confirm whether your child is anaemic.

The most common cause is lack of iron or vitamins in the diet, and medicines recommended by your doctor will replace these.

POISONING

Children are inquisitive, and accidental poisoning is common. Drugs and medicines, household chemicals such as bleaches and detergents, and berries or seeds from outside, are the most common cause of problems.

Medicines are probably the most dangerous, and are the main cause of death amongst the two dozen or so children who die each year from poisoning in this country. Paracetamol, antidepressants, aspirin and iron tablets are particularly dangerous.

IF YOUR CHILD HAS TAKEN MORE THAN THE RECOMMENDED DOSE OF ANY DRUG then CHECK WITH YOUR DOCTOR or local CASUALTY DEPARTMENT. If the overdose is only small, and you are sure of the precise amount taken, this may simply involve a telephone call for advice. Often it isn't possible to be so sure and, if in doubt, TAKE YOUR CHILD TO CASUALTY.

If the drug is **paracetamol**, **digoxin** (used to treat heart conditions, usually in older people), **aspirin**, **iron** or an **antidepressant**, then GO STRAIGHT TO CASUALTY, as these can be particularly dangerous.

POISONING WITH BERRIES, SEEDS OR HOUSEHOLD CHEMICALS may be less serious, although some of these can be very dangerous indeed. Powerful bleaches, petrol, turpentine and paraffin may cause damage to the oesophagus (gullet) or lungs.

GUIDANCE
Treatment of poisoning often means making your child sick to clear the poison from the stomach. As a general rule, this is a job for TRAINED MEDICAL STAFF, ideally in your LOCAL CASUALTY DEPARTMENT.

❖   ❖   ❖

If your child has taken poison and you can't get him or her to casualty within the next hour, then you may have to make the child sick yourself. ALWAYS CHECK WITH A DOCTOR **before** you do this; vomiting is actually dangerous with some poisons, such as the household chemicals mentioned above. Another danger is that the child will breathe-in the vomit. This is a risk if he or she is very drowsy or unconscious, in which case you shouldn't try to cause vomiting.

❖   ❖   ❖

The best way to cause vomiting is with a dose of **syrup of ipecacuanha**, available from the chemist. If you live in an isolated or remote area, it is a good idea to have this around, just in case. Poking the back of the child's throat with your finger is a last resort, and may well injure your finger as well as his or her throat.

❖   ❖   ❖

Drinking plenty of fluids, especially milk, will help to dilute the poison and will also make vomiting easier. Milk is especially important for poisoning with household chemicals, where vomiting is dangerous. Give your child a drink of milk while you are waiting to reach medical help.

❖   ❖   ❖   ❖   ❖

PREVENTION
Prevention of poisoning accidents is better than cure. Casualty departments in this country still see around 40 000 children every year with poisoning.

Keep all medicines and chemicals safely locked away and out of reach. Your health visitor will be able to give you more specific advice.

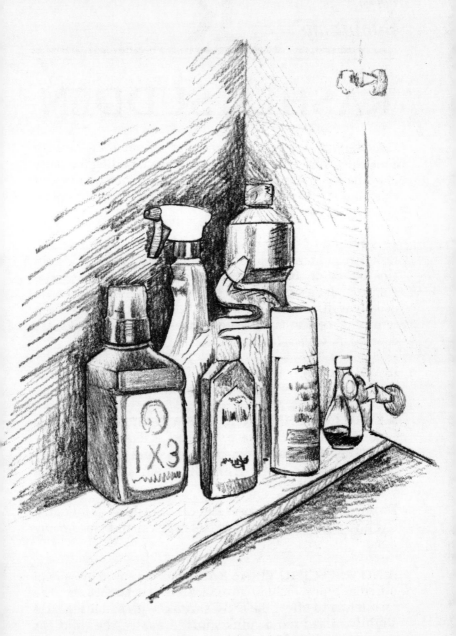

Keep all medicines and chemicals safely locked away and out of reach

RASHES, SUDDEN

Sometimes you or your doctor can be certain of the cause of a rash after one glance. But far more often, finding the cause is a matter of careful detective work, examination and checking symptoms. Even then your doctor might not be able to give you a precise cause.

This section of the book can't enable you to diagnose any rash that suddenly appears on your child's body, but it does aim to provide some pointers that might help to find what is going on. It describes rashes that appear in children who are usually well, and not prone to rashes. Skin rashes that keep returning, or that last for more than a couple of weeks, are covered in *Rashes, long-term*.

IF YOUR CHILD HAS A FEW SEPARATE SPOTS rather than a rash then see *Spots, non itchy* and *Spots, itchy*.

A RASH IN A CHILD WHO HAS A TEMPERATURE or is generally unwell, flu-like, or off food, is likely to be caused by a **virus infection**. Sometimes the child may have very few symptoms apart from the rash, and may seem remarkably well.

Dozens of different viruses can cause rashes. Although a few give characteristic patterns that you can recognise, many don't.

A NON SPECIFIC VIRAL RASH can be caused by several different types, including **coxsackie** and **echo viruses**. The rash tends to affect the child's trunk, with small separate slightly raised red or pink spots. Usually, the child has symptoms of a cold or mild stomach upset but is quite well in himself or herself. The rash generally fades after three or four days.

MEASLES RASH usually starts on the child's face and behind the ears, spreading downwards over the trunk, arms and legs. The spots are red and blotchy, and tend to join up and run into one another – unlike a non specific rash.

Children with measles are usually very poorly; if your child is in good health with his or her rash then the diagnosis almost certainly isn't measles.

With measles, symptoms of a cold often appear a couple of days before the rash appears. The child may have sore, red eyes and white spots (**Koplik's spots**) on the inside of the mouth. As the rash starts to fade after a few days it may become dry and scaly.

GUIDANCE
Treatment of measles simply means keeping your child cool and comfortable with drinks and paracetamol (see dosage, page 11).

❖   ❖   ❖

Complications are relatively common, so SEE YOUR DOCTOR if your child develops earache (possibility of ear infection), a bad cough or shortness of breath (pneumonia) or signs of meningitis (see *Neck, stiff or painful*; possibility of brain inflammation).

GERMAN MEASLES (RUBELLA) may produce a similar rash to measles, but mainly on the child's trunk. The child will be quite well and have symptoms of a cold and maybe enlarged glands in the neck, particularly at the back. The rubella rash may also look quite similar to a non specific rash and, for this reason, it isn't usually possible to be sure of the diagnosis simply by looking. SEE YOUR DOCTOR; doctors tend to play safe and recommend rubella precautions (keeping away from pregnant women and other children) until any rash has cleared.

GUIDANCE
Complications virtually never occur, although adolescent girls may experience joint pains.

209

❖   ❖   ❖

Treatment is rest, drinks and paracetamol (see dosage, page 11).

CHICKENPOX does usually produce an easily recognisable rash. Small clear blisters, like drops of water, appear on the trunk and burst after a couple of days to form scabs. The moist scabs gradually dry and heal over about seven days. New spots keep forming for the first three or four days, so altogether it takes around ten days for all the spots to dry. The spots are itchy although the child is otherwise quite well.

GUIDANCE
The child should be kept away from other children until all the spots have dried.

❖   ❖   ❖

Any fever and headache can be treated with paracetamol (see dosage, page 11).

❖   ❖   ❖

Calamine lotion on to the skin, or promethazine syrup by mouth (from the chemist – an antihistamine which may make your child drowsy) will help to control the itching.

❖   ❖   ❖

Complications are very rare.

ROSEOLA INFANTUM is common, despite the fact that few people have heard of it. The child may be quite ill with a fever and cold symptoms for two or three days before the rash suddenly appears. The rash is similar to the non specific rash described above, but as soon as the rash appears, the fever drops and the child becomes much better; this usually gives away the diagnosis. The cause is a virus infection.

GUIDANCE
Treatment simply means treating fever with paracetamol (see dosage, page 11).

SCARLET FEVER isn't actually a virus infection. It is caused by a **bacterium, the streptococcus**, that causes some sore throats. The child develops a sore throat with swollen, inflamed tonsils often flecked with spots of pus (see *Throat, sore*).

The rash appears as tiny red spots on the trunk together with flushed cheeks and a paler area around the mouth. The tongue may be sore or white and coated, and the child may be quite ill. SEE YOUR DOCTOR.

DOCTOR'S TREATMENT
Although complications are very rare, nowadays, they do include ear infections and, rarely, kidney or heart damage.

For this reason your doctor will treat scarlet fever with penicillin, to which the streptococcus bug is sensitive.

MMR VACCINE may occasionally produce a non specific rash after about a week (see *Immunisation reactions*).

A RASH OF SMALL PURPLE BLOTCHES may be a sign of meningitis (see *Neck, stiff*) and should be taken seriously, so SEE YOUR DOCTOR.

The child is likely to be quite, or very, ill (see *Ill – should your child see the doctor?*).

TINY PURPLE SPOTS AROUND THE EYES OR OVER THE FACE may be the result of a prolonged and severe bout of coughing, or straining on the loo.

The child strains so hard that tiny blood vessels burst in the skin of his or her face.

These spots are harmless, although may take a couple of weeks to disappear.

ALLERGY is the other most likely cause of a sudden rash. The child may be reacting to something with which his or her skin is in contact. This may produce a rash in one or two places (for example, contact with nickel in clothing fastenings, or with plants) or be more widespread (for example, traces of washing powder on clothes). Or the allergy may be due to something the child has swallowed. Drugs such as antibiotics are often to blame, although food colourings, flavourings, shellfish and other foods are all notorious too.

An allergic rash is usually similar to the non specific rash described earlier in this section, although it may appear more dry and itchy, as with eczema (see *Rashes, long-term*). It often affects most of the body. Usually the rash will fade within a few days, once the cause has been removed.

Finding out just what did trigger the rash sometimes involves a great deal of detective work, and often isn't possible even then – the rash simply appears and disappears again mysteriously several days later.

GUIDANCE
The child isn't generally unwell and shouldn't have a fever although the rash may itch slightly.

❖   ❖   ❖

Swelling around the eyes, noisy breathing or wheezing may be a sign of a more serious allergy and you should SEE YOUR DOCTOR IMMEDIATELY.

❖   ❖   ❖

Treatment means finding and removing the cause if possible.

❖   ❖   ❖

Antihistamines from the chemist (chlorpheniramine, which may cause drowsiness, or terfenadine which won't) will help to reduce the rash.

AN ITCHY RASH WHICH COMES AND GOES VERY QUICKLY, appearing and disappearing or moving around the body from one place to the other over hours or even minutes, is likely to be **urticaria** (see *Itching anywhere*).

A VERY ITCHY RASH raises the possibility of **scabies** (see *Itching anywhere*).

NAPPY RASH is described in *Nappy rash*.

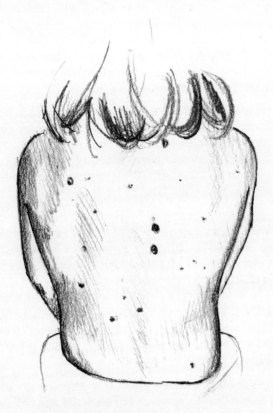

Chickenpox spots mainly affect the trunk and the face

213

RASHES, LONG-TERM

This section describes some of the common rashes which last longer than a couple of weeks, or which keep returning. Occasionally, a sudden, short-term rash (see *Rashes, sudden*) may persist for a couple of weeks but will generally fade shortly afterwards.

ECZEMA (DERMATITIS) is the most common form of long-term rash. **Eczema** and **dermatitis** are two words meaning **exactly the same thing**.

Eczema means dry, inflamed skin. At first the skin becomes dry, and in mild cases this may be as far as it goes. In more severe cases the skin becomes red and scaly, and also very itchy. The cause is unknown, although eczema is often passed in families, together with a tendency to hay fever or asthma.

Milk allergy may sometimes be partly to blame, and some children with eczema do get worse if they eat or drink dairy products. Breast-feeding for as long as possible, while keeping your baby off all other forms of milk, may reduce the child's risk of developing eczema later on.

ECZEMA IN BABIES usually affects the cheeks, behind the ears and the body. Often the scalp is affected too, with cradle cap (see *Cradle cap and dandruff*), which is part of the same problem.

Usually this form of eczema gradually improves, and about half of all babies have grown out of it by the age of five years and most by the age of ten. In a few children it does persist.

ECZEMA IN TODDLERS AND OLDER CHILDREN is similar to eczema in adults. It particularly affects the front of the elbows, the back of the knees, the neck, face and wrists.

INFECTED ECZEMA is quite common. Bacteria that normally live quite harmlessly on the skin, can infect the inflamed, broken skin of eczema particularly if the child scratches it. Infected eczema may become weepy with a yellow crust and enlarged glands in the area, or there may not be much sign of infection.

Suspect infection if your child's eczema is spreading rapidly despite your normal treatment. SEE YOUR DOCTOR who will treat infection with antibiotics applied to the skin or taken by mouth.

DOCTOR'S TREATMENT
Treatment of eczema means keeping it under control. This is the best you can aim for; although eczema in small children usually disappears eventually, there is no cure that can actually get rid of the rash for ever. But modern treatments will virtually always keep the symptoms at bay.

❖　　　❖　　　❖

You and your doctor will need to work out the treatment that suits your child best, and will need to change it from time to time as the eczema flares up or improves.

❖　　　❖　　　❖

As a general rule, avoid soap, bath bubbles or baby bath liquids, which dry the skin. Use a moisturising cream such as aqueous cream from the chemist to keep dry skin moist.

❖　　　❖　　　❖

Your doctor may suggest an emollient (moisturising) agent such as emulsifying ointment to add to your child's bath or to use as a moisturising soap substitute.

❖　　　❖　　　❖

Steroid creams, such as hydrocortisone or other, stronger, forms are invaluable to control more severe eczema, but you

215

should use them only UNDER YOUR DOCTOR'S GUIDANCE.

PSORIASIS sometimes affects young children around the age of 10 years, although it is most common in adults. It may be passed in families. Psoriasis usually appears as a round or oval patch of purple or pink skin covered with silvery flaking scales. It tends to affect the back of the elbows and the front of the knees, unlike eczema. Generally, it doesn't itch as much as eczema.

Psoriasis is completely different from eczema, although the two may sometimes look similar. The cause is an increase in the rate at which skin cells grow and flake off – all skin cells do this, but in psoriasis they do it many times faster than normal.

As with eczema, **treatment** means using creams and medicines to keep the rash under control rather than to provide a permanent cure.

IMPETIGO is a skin infection usually with the bacterium **staphylococcus aureus**, which also causes boils. It usually affects the face, particularly around the nose and mouth, and the hands.

It starts as a small red patch which steadily spreads. The red skin becomes weepy and eventually covered with a yellow crust of dried pus.

GUIDANCE
Impetigo may last for weeks or months without treatment. It is infectious and your child shouldn't go to school or mix with other children until it has cleared.

❖   ❖   ❖

SEE YOUR DOCTOR: a course of antibiotics, either taken by mouth or applied to the rash, should provide a rapid cure.

❖   ❖   ❖

Impetigo that keeps coming back may mean that one member of the family is carrying the staphylococcus, and needs to be treated in the same way as do recurrent boils (see *Boils*).

RINGWORM is a **fungus infection** of the skin. It has nothing to do with worms or rings. The name arises because a patch of ringworm looks circular (the ring) with a sharp red edge (like a worm). The skin in the centre of the patch may appear quite normal, with the skin around the edge being red and scaly. Ringworm is usually fairly itchy.

Ringworm may affect any part of the body, arms or legs. Other forms of the ringworm fungus affect other areas, particularly the groin.

GUIDANCE
Treatment of ringworm is with an anti-fungal cream from your doctor or available without prescription from your chemist.

❖　　　❖　　　❖

Although you may need to persevere for several weeks, the ringworm should clear completely.

❖　　　❖　　　❖

Other children may catch ringworm by touching the affected area, so this should be covered up with a dressing if it is on an exposed part of your child's body.

RINGWORM OF THE SCALP causes an itchy scaly scalp with patches of hair loss (see *Hair loss*).

ATHLETE'S FOOT is caused by **ringworm of the feet**. It appears between the toes, occasionally on the sole of the foot itself. The skin becomes red and scaly but if sweat, and constant rubbing together of the toes, keeps it moist and irritated, it may become soggy, swollen and smelly.

The fungus thrives in warm damp conditions such as shower room or changing room floors, and is often passed on in this way.

GUIDANCE
Treatment of athlete's foot means keeping your child's feet dry, using shoes which allow the feet to breathe (sandals, canvas or leather shoes are best; trainers often seem to make the problem worse) and using an anti-fungal cream from your chemist.

❖   ❖   ❖

Athlete's foot powders may help to prevent the problem from returning, but aren't likely to be enough to get rid of it.

PSORIASIS   ECZEMA

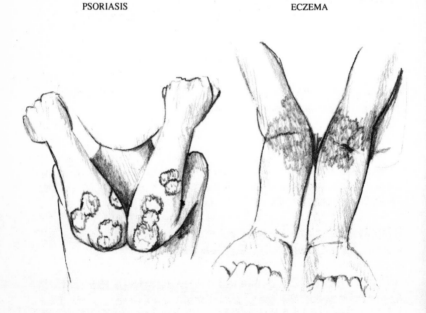

Psoriasis particularly affects knees, elbows and scalp
Eczema tends to affect different areas at different ages

READING AND SCHOOL PROBLEMS

Variations in the rate at which they learn to read, and a reluctance at one stage or another to go to school, are normal among children of all ages. Occasionally, the problem may need professional help.

As many as one in ten children starting secondary school have difficulty reading. Often there is a combination of reasons to do with the child's abilities, his or her teaching at school and encouragement at home. But a few children really do seem to find reading far harder than their intelligence, schooling and other abilities suggest that they should.

DYSLEXIA is the name given to this problem although many experts nowadays prefer the term **specific reading retardation**. It probably affects around two or three per cent of school children, boys more than girls, and may occasionally run in a family. The cause isn't known, although some of these children seem to be unusually clumsy too, and dyslexia may have a similar cause to clumsiness (see *Clumsiness*).

Truly dyslexic children may find great difficulty in writing as well as reading. They may form letters backwards, write whole words backwards, or find spelling impossible.

GUIDANCE
The **diagnosis of dyslexia** depends on an expert assessment, usually from an educational psychologist. Your doctor or, more usually, your child's school, should be able to arrange this.

❖　　　❖　　　❖

Not all doctors or psychologists agree about the diagnosis, or even whether the condition exists at all.

SCHOOL PROBLEMS are common, and many children complain from time to time of feeling ill on Monday mornings in the hope of avoiding the day at school.

SCHOOL REFUSAL means that this has become a real problem, and the child is actually missing a substantial amount of school.

True school refusal is quite rare, and it is different from truancy. Truant children are simply choosing to avoid school for antisocial reasons, preferring to do something else. School refusers are generally very anxious about one or more aspects of school. This anxiety may develop into a true phobia where the child simply can't face up to his or her fears.

School refusal starts gradually, with symptoms such as headaches or sickness that appear increasingly frequently at the beginning of each school day. The child starts to miss more and more school. He or she may be afraid of bullying, other children, a particular teacher, the school toilets, dangers on the journey to school, or a combination of factors. Sometimes teachers will send the child home once he or she has arrived at school, because of various symptoms.

GUIDANCE
Usually these fears can be spotted and nipped in the bud by parents. If school refusal does become a problem that you can't handle, then you may need help from the school, your health visitor or doctor, or an educational psychologist.

SOLVENT ABUSE is also known as **glue sniffing**, although many other volatile chemicals such as petrol and dry-cleaning fluid are used too. Behaviour problems, usually antisocial or even criminal, are common in youngsters who indulge.

The child may breathe the fumes directly from the tube or bottle, or first pour the chemical into a plastic bag and put this over his or her mouth and nose. Some children have died through suffocation in this way, and others from shock caused by releasing sprays or aerosols into the throat (see *Paleness* for a description of **shock**).

The sensation is immediate and is similar to being drunk on alcohol. The child may become unsteady on his or her feet with blurred vision and even visual hallucinations, seeing things that aren't there. These feelings usually disappear almost as quickly as they began once the child stops sniffing, although he or she may be left with a mild headache.

GUIDANCE
Solvent abuse can be difficult to spot. Chemical smells on the child's breath or in his or her room, empty containers, episodes of odd behaviour, or a rash around the chin and bridge of the nose where the plastic bag rubs, may be telltale signs.

SEE YOUR DOCTOR, who should be able to tell you where to go for help.

SLEEP PROBLEMS

Most parents of babies and young children expect a few disturbed nights. But there is great variation in what different parents regard as normal, and also in the actual sleeping patterns of different children. Sometimes this becomes a problem.

On average, about one-third of three-month-old babies wake at night. One in five of two-year-olds, and one in ten of all four-year-olds, still wake regularly. For many children a fitful pattern of sleep is quite normal. Children, like adults, also seem to vary in the amount of sleep they actually need. Usually, a calmer night-time sleeping pattern appears after the age of five years.

With patience and persistence, you can almost always change your child's sleeping pattern to one which is less disruptive to you and the family. This section can only give a few pointers to the kind of tactics you may need to use. All children are different, and if you do want to change the way your child behaves at night, then you will have to decide what will work best for him or her. Your health visitor is trained and experienced in sleep problems, and should be able to help you to choose your approach.

NIGHTMARES, NIGHT TERRORS AND SLEEP-WALKING worry some older children at night (see *Nightmares, night terrors and sleepwalking*).

WAKING EARLY IN THE MORNING is so common as to be accepted as normal by many parents.

A later bedtime is an obvious way around the problem, but this doesn't, in fact, help as often as it should. Some children wake because they are hungry, and a drink or a biscuit by the bed will sometimes settle the child for a while. Older children may obey if they are told not to disturb their parents before a certain time, or until an alarm clock has gone off.

CHILDREN WHO MAKE A FUSS ABOUT GOING TO BED may be afraid of the dark, or monsters under the bed. A night light or a favourite toy may provide some comfort.

Often the problem is simply that the child isn't tired. Try waking him or her earlier in the morning, or moving bedtime back a few minutes every night until things improve. Once you have found a bedtime that seems to work, insist your child sticks to it.

CHILDREN WHO CLIMB INTO THEIR PARENTS' BED can disrupt a marriage as well as your sleep.

An exhausting few nights of taking the child back to his or her bed every time will usually break the cycle, but you do have to stick with it. Sometimes it is easier if smaller children have their cot in your room for a while.

CHILDREN WHO KEEP WAKING AT NIGHT are a common problem. Although it is easier to give the child what he or she wants – a drink, food, or a playtime – in order to get yourself back to bed as soon as possible, this may in fact prolong the problem. In effect, you are teaching your child that waking at night is rewarded in this way.

GUIDANCE
Leaving babies or young children to cry themselves to sleep is an old remedy that you will probably be advised to try. It does work; within a few nights your baby will almost certainly stop waking. And it doesn't carry any risk of damage or psychological trauma to the child. But it takes nerves of steel on your part! Many parents find that listening to their own child screaming and sobbing is simply too much to bear; and for this method to work, you mustn't give in and go to your child.

223

If you do decide to try this, it is best to discuss it with your health visitor first.

❖　　❖　　❖

Another method is simply to go to your child without turning on the light, without offering food or a drink, or doing anything else that suggests that fun and attention is on offer. Reassure him or her that you are there, and go back to bed once your child has started to settle.

You may be back again within a few minutes, and probably many times over the next few exhausting nights, but your child will get the message that night-time is for sleeping, and should start to settle on his or her own.

❖　　❖　　❖

When these methods don't work, it is possible that you haven't been able to stick rigorously enough to the method you have chosen, or there may be another method which would suit your child better.

Talk the problem over with your health visitor before trying again.

SNORING AND BLOCKED NOSE

Snoring is surprisingly common in children. Usually the child's nose will be partly or completely blocked during the day as well, and this may affect his or her speech.

ENLARGED ADENOIDS are the most common cause of snoring in children. The adenoids are glands at the back of the nose. Like other glands in this area (the tonsils and lymph glands in the neck – see *Lumps in the neck*), they form part of the body's immune system which fights infection. Colds and sore throats cause the adenoids to swell as they help prevent the spread of infection.

Most children suffer repeated coughs and colds, and sometimes the adenoids become permanently swollen as a result. This causes a blockage at the back of the nose. The blockage isn't usually total, and the child can breathe through his or her nose even though this may be quite noisy. But lying flat worsens the blockage, especially during sleep when the muscles in the child's throat are relaxed, and causes snoring as the child breathes in.

Permanently swollen adenoids can affect the child's speech too. In order to produce sounds such as 'm' and 'n' properly, the child needs to be able to force air out through his or her nose. Enlarged adenoids will prevent this.

Badly swollen adenoids may stop the child breathing through his or her nose by day as well as night, causing a permanently open and dry mouth. Eating might be difficult as well as unpleasant to watch, as the child tries to breathe through his or her mouth at the same time as chewing food.

GUIDANCE
Treatment for permanently enlarged adenoids may not be necessary, since they start to shrink after the age of about

225

seven years, and have usually virtually disappeared by adult life.

✦　　✦　　✦

Adenoids that are causing severe snoring or speech problems, or that are causing recurrent ear infections by blocking the **eustachian tube** which drains the middle ear (see *Pain or discharge in the ear*) may need to be removed by surgery, so SEE YOUR DOCTOR in such cases.

SNORING OR A BLOCKED NOSE DURING A COLD is caused by swollen adenoids as well as swelling of the rest of the nose and throat, and a build up of excess mucus.

Decongestant nose drops and a steamy atmosphere may help, and the problem should disappear within a week or two.

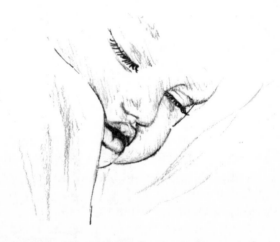

Badly swollen adenoids may block the nose and cause a permanently open, dry mouth

A BLOCKED NOSE WITHOUT MUCH SNORING may be caused by allergy (see *Hay fever and nose allergies*), a cold or a foreign object in the nostril (see *Foreign objects*).

❖   ❖   ❖   ❖   ❖

HOME TREATMENT
General treatment for snoring may mean keeping a check on your child's weight. Older children and adults who are very overweight are more prone to snoring as the muscles in their throats seem to be more floppy. Losing the excess weight generally seems to cure the problem.

❖   ❖   ❖

Otherwise a steamy atmosphere at night (see *Cough, hoarse and croupy*) may help.

❖   ❖   ❖

If you can stop your child from sleeping on his or her back, then the snoring will often disappear too – but this isn't easy, as children tend to roll over in bed however well they are propped up.

SPEECH PROBLEMS AND STAMMERING

Different children may learn to speak at very different rates but on average most babies will start to babble at around six months of age. The babbling gradually changes into sounds such as 'da-da' and 'mum-mum' by about nine months, although usually still without any meaning. The child starts to use single words with meaning, such as 'mummy' or 'cat', at about one year, and is able to understand and obey simple commands such as 'give it to mummy'.

By the age of two years, most children are putting two, three or more words together in simple sentences. By the age of three-and-a-half years, they are regular chatterboxes, making sentences which are full and mostly grammatically correct.

SLOW DEVELOPMENT OF SPEECH may have several causes, although the commonest and most important is **poor hearing**. Children need to hear the full range of sounds made by normal speech in order to learn proper speech themselves. Hearing loss is quite common (see *Hearing problems*), usually caused by fluid inside the ear. Although this may only cause a partial degree of deafness, it tends to prevent the child from hearing consonant sounds, such as 's' and 'k', which are vital for the development of speech.

Children also need constant attention, stimulation and talking to in order to learn speech and language themselves. Emotionally deprived children tend to be slow in learning to talk, whereas children who have been constantly stimulated develop faster.

More rarely, mental retardation or autism may cause very great delay in the development of speech.

GUIDANCE
As a general rule, you should SEE YOUR DOCTOR if your child's speech development falls behind the pattern described at the beginning of this section, although there is a considerable variation in the normal, and your doctor may simply reassure you that all seems well.

CHILDREN WHO KNOW WHAT THEY WANT TO SAY BUT CAN'T PRONOUNCE THE WORDS PROPERLY are very common and, in fact, this is a normal stage of development around the age of three years. Strangers may find your child difficult or impossible to understand at times, but most of the time you are able to make sense of what he or she is saying.

Provided that the child's hearing is normal (see *Hearing problems*), his or her speech should soon become intelligible. Often, starting nursery or playgroup helps enormously, as the child starts to socialise with others and learns to make himself or herself understood.

GUIDANCE
Almost always your child's speech will become clear within a short time, but SEE YOUR DOCTOR if

◆ you can't understand what he or she is saying most of the time by the age of three years, OR

◆ others can't understand your child by the age of four years, OR

◆ you suspect your child may not be hearing properly (see *Hearing problems*).

PHYSICAL CAUSES OF UNINTELLIGIBLE SPEECH are much more rare. You should SEE YOUR DOCTOR.

A **tongue tie**, where the **frenulum** (the piece of membrane joining the tongue to the base of the mouth) is too tight, was often diagnosed in the past, but nowadays most doctors don't believe that it often affects speech. If necessary, treatment is simply by cutting the frenulum.

Children with cleft palates, blocked noses (see *Snoring and blocked nose*), or cerebral palsy (brain damage at birth) may be unable to pronounce some sounds properly.

STAMMERING is another problem that is so common as to be in fact a normal part of speech development. Many children stammer around the ages of three and four years, when they are learning many new words faster than they can pronounce them.

At first, the child simply repeats the sound at the start of the word over and over again before pronouncing it in some form or another. Occasionally, the stammering develops further; the child's speech grinds to a halt once he or she encounters a tricky word, and the child may start to avoid words that cause problems. Probably about one in twenty-five children are affected like this, and may find problems with school as well as teasing from other children.

GUIDANCE
Since nearly all children grow out of their phase of stammering, there is no need for any treatment unless your child is over six years of age, or is having problems at school because of the stammer.

❖   ❖   ❖

Treatment usually means a course of speech therapy. Otherwise you can safely wait for things to improve.

❖   ❖   ❖

Don't draw attention to your child's stammering, or force him or her to repeat difficult words, as this is simply likely to draw attention to the problem and make matters worse.

SPINE, CURVED

The spine or backbone is made from a row of 24 bones, the vertebrae, connected by tough discs of gristle and jelly. Seen from the side, the spine is S-shaped, but viewed from the back it should be straight. Sometimes, an abnormal curvature of the spine can lead to problems if it isn't spotted and treated in time.

A CURVATURE FROM FRONT TO BACK, that is only obvious from looking at the side, is called a **kyphosis**.

Kyphosis is quite rare in children, and is usually the result of damage to the vertebrae from infection or an injury.

A SPINE THAT IS CURVED FROM SIDE TO SIDE, so that the curvature is obvious from looking at the back, is called a **scoliosis**.

Scoliosis is much more common, and up to four in every thousand children need treatment for it. Usually it appears around the age of 10 or 12 years. Although it doesn't cause the child any pain or other symptoms, if he or she stands stripped to the waist and facing away from you, then you will see that the spine is curved to one side.

The curve may affect any part of the spine. In fact there are usually at least two separate curves, in opposite directions; the child has developed the second curve in order to counteract the effect of the first so as to keep his or her head straight.

As the scoliosis develops, a hump starts to appear alongside the curve, on the side that lies on the outside of the curve. The hump appears because the vertebrae in the curve become twisted too. The ribs, that are attached to the vertebrae, become pushed out and prominent in that area to form a hump.

This is by far the most common type of scoliosis; it simply seems to develop, and nobody really knows why. More rarely, children are born with scoliosis caused by an abnormally developed vertebrae or they develop it after damage to the muscles supporting the spine, for example through infection with polio. If the child's legs aren't the same length then he or she will curve the spine in order to keep the upper body and head straight; this is called a **compensatory scoliosis**.

SCOLIOSIS IN BABIES is very rare but does sometimes occur. As with older children, the cause isn't known.

❖   ❖   ❖   ❖   ❖

GUIDANCE
What may happen to your child's scoliosis is generally a matter for expert assessment. Many cases of scoliosis simply get better without any treatment.

❖   ❖   ❖

As a general rule, scoliosis affecting the **lumbar spine** (the lower part of the spine) is more likely to recover than scoliosis of the **thoracic spine** (attached to the rib-cage), and the later the scoliosis starts the better.

❖   ❖   ❖

Scoliosis that disappears completely when your child bends forward, is almost certain to cause no problems.

DOCTOR'S TREATMENT
More severe scoliosis may continue to develop if it isn't treated, resulting in permanent deformity and even breathing difficulty as the lungs become squashed inside the cramped rib-cage.

❖   ❖   ❖

SEE A DOCTOR if you have **any suspicion that your child has scoliosis**, unless you are **absolutely sure** that the curve disappears totally on bending forward.

✧   ✧   ✧

If treatment is necessary, then this might mean wearing a special brace or, in older children and adolescents, surgery to straighten the spine.

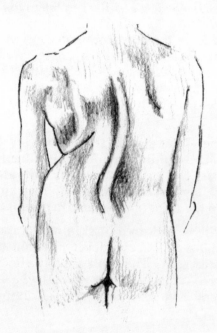

Scoliosis means a spine that is curved from side to side

SPOTS, ITCHY

Just when a group of spots becomes a rash is a matter of opinion, but this section covers the common causes of a few separate itchy spots that suddenly appear. For other causes of itching, or more widespread spots and rashes, see *Itching anywhere*; *Rashes, sudden*; and *Rashes, long-term*.

INSECT BITES are the most common causes of a crop of itchy spots. The spots are actually an **allergic reaction to the bites**, and some people are much less sensitive to them than others. This explains why some people will develop huge itchy spots after insect bites, whereas others will have little or no reaction.

Although babies don't usually seem to be very sensitive to insect bites, older children are often quite badly affected. After a few years, this sensitivity usually fades and the child becomes much less prone to dozens of itchy bumps every summer (when the crops of spots tend to return).

An itchy white raised area of skin may appear within minutes of an insect bite, and develop within a few hours into a raised red spot. The spots usually affect arms and legs, and tend to occur in groups or lines where one insect has taken several bites in succession. They disappear after a week or two.

GUIDANCE
Finding the insect responsible isn't always easy, and may take some detective work. **Ants or flying insects** are most likely if the bites occurred outside.

❖   ❖   ❖

Fleas are a common cause of bites indoors, usually from a dog or cat (human fleas are very rare nowadays). Getting rid of fleas may involve treating carpet and soft furnishings as well as your pet.

❖   ❖   ❖

Pets can also carry tiny **mites** which can bite humans; they can be treated but you should have your pet examined by a vet first.

❖   ❖   ❖

Bed bugs may live in furniture or in nooks and crannies around the room as well as in the bed itself, and so they are often difficult to spot by day. They bite at night, usually causing groups of spots on exposed areas of skin such as the child's face and hands.

❖   ❖   ❖

Several members of the family may be affected by bites. However, sometimes just one child seems to get spots, and this doesn't mean that insect bites aren't to blame.

HOME TREATMENT
Treatment of insect bites means controlling the itching with antihistamines by mouth (promethazine or chlorpheniramine, available from your chemist), or calamine lotion or hydrocortisone cream applied to the skin.

❖   ❖   ❖

Insect repellents might be useful for children who suffer at a particular time of year, or when going abroad on holiday.

❖   ❖   ❖

Pet shops and general stores usually sell powders and sprays to clear fleas and mites from carpets and furnishings, as well as preparations to treat your pets.

❖   ❖   ❖

If the bites still return, then SEE YOUR DOCTOR to confirm the diagnosis; it might then be necessary to call in professional help in clearing the infestation, from your local council or a private specialist contractor.

STINGS are usually caused by wasps or bees. Bee stings may remain in the skin afterwards; if you can see the sting, try to remove it by scraping with the flat blade of a knife or a fingernail. Don't use tweezers, as this is likely to cause the sting to break off.

HOME TREATMENT
Meat tenderiser, if you have it in your kitchen, is a useful and often immediate remedy for the pain. Dilute it with water (one part tenderiser to five parts water) and apply it to the sting.

❖   ❖   ❖

Otherwise, putting **vinegar** on to **wasp stings**, and **bicarbonate** on to **bee stings**, is a tried and trusted remedy.

❖   ❖   ❖

An ice cube held on to the affected area will help to reduce pain and swelling too. Paracetamol is also useful for pain (see dosage, page 11).

STINGS INSIDE THE MOUTH are unusual, but can cause severe swelling of the tongue or throat with the danger of choking.

SEE A DOCTOR AT ONCE if you think that your child has been stung inside the mouth. DIAL 999 or TAKE THE CHILD STRAIGHT TO CASUALTY if there is any sign of difficult breathing (see *Breathing, noisy or difficult*).

AN ALLERGIC REACTION TO A STING, where a child reacts badly, with a large red swollen area around the sting, should be treated in the same way as for an allergic reaction to an insect bite (see above).

Very rarely, a child may have a severe allergic reaction to a sting with breathing difficulty, collapse and even unconsciousness. This is an **emergency** and you should DIAL 999 FOR IMMEDIATE MEDICAL ATTENTION.

CHICKENPOX SPOTS are probably the only spots that could be confused with insect bites. When chickenpox spots first appear they are itchy, although usually more and more spots quickly appear over the body. The spots form blisters and then burst to leave a scab (see **Chickenpox** in *Rashes, sudden*).

SCABIES is a mite which burrows under the skin to produce very itchy spots, often in the armpits, groin or between the fingers. Usually the spots are flatter and more itchy than insect bites, and you may see a tiny burrow under the skin leading from the spot (see **Scabies** in *Itching anywhere*).

PIMPLES AND ACNE SPOTS may occasionally be sore or slightly itchy (see *Spots, non itchy*).

SPOTS, NON ITCHY

ACNE AND PIMPLES are the most common cause of spots. They can affect young children and even babies, but usually start around the age of 12 to 14 years, and most teenagers are affected to some extent.

Acne is caused by a problem with the sweat glands in the skin. These glands produce sweat, and are partly under the control of the **sex hormone, testosterone**, in the bloodstream. The surge in the level of sex hormones that starts at puberty often seems to be the trigger for the glands to malfunction and develop acne.

Teenagers with bad acne don't necessarily produce more hormone than others, but their sweat glands seem unusually sensitive to its effects. **Infection of the sweat gland**, and **blockage of the pore** – the opening of the sweat gland onto the surface of the skin – follow, and acne develops.

Usually the spots affect the face and the upper part of the chest, shoulders and back. The spots are red and raised, and sometimes form fluid-filled cysts. Often, there will be **blackheads**, tiny black dots in the skin which are in fact the blocked pores of sweat glands.

Severe acne, after a year or two, may leave permanent scarring. Eventually, the acne almost always clears by the mid-twenties, although rarely can last into the thirties or beyond.

GUIDANCE
Treatment of acne is usually quite effective, although it may involve a combination of methods. Contrary to general belief diet doesn't often seem to make much difference, and avoiding fatty food or chocolate isn't likely to help.

❖ ❖ ❖

Regular washing with soap and water, to keep the skin pores clear, is important; sometimes a bactericidal soap, available from the chemist, helps to reduce the number of bacteria on your child's skin.

❖   ❖   ❖

More powerful skin cleansers, such as **benzoyl peroxide**, are also available without prescription; they help to remove the dead surface skin layer and so keep the pores clear. Be prepared for them to inflame the skin at first. After a couple of weeks of sore, red, blotchy skin that looks worse than ever, your child's complexion should start to improve.

❖   ❖   ❖

Sunlight, although potentially harmful to the skin in large doses, usually helps to clear acne.

DOCTOR'S TREATMENT
SEE YOUR DOCTOR if the above measures aren't enough. He or she may prescribe antibiotics, either as tablets by mouth or as cream or lotion to apply to the skin, to be used for a long period of time to control the infection that helps trigger acne.

❖   ❖   ❖

Older teenage girls with severe acne may be prescribed a special form of the pill containing a hormone which counteracts the effects of the sex hormone testosterone on the skin.

❖   ❖   ❖

A more powerful drug, **isotretinoin**, is usually only available from hospital specialists for treating **severe acne**. It can cause liver damage, and is extremely dangerous to an unborn child – which is why it isn't generally used for girls or women who could possibly become pregnant, unless they are using reliable contraception.

OTHER CAUSES OF NON ITCHY SPOTS may include: boils (see *Boils*); a rash caused by allergy or infection if there are several spots over a wide area (see *Rashes, sudden*); or erythema nodosum (see below).

ERYTHEMA NODOSUM means one or more red lumps which usually appear over the shins or sometimes the forearms. They are tender and may be quite large, two centimetres or more across. The lumps may be raised like small domes, or may be quite flat. They usually disappear after a few weeks.

There are several possible causes including infections, drugs and bowel disorders.

ALWAYS SEE YOUR DOCTOR if you suspect erythema nodosum; although most causes are harmless, a few, such as colitis or bowel inflammation, are potentially serious and should be checked for.

WARTS are small, hard, raised spots which may occur in crops or clusters. **Molluscum** is a kind of wart which produces pink, domed spots often with a small dimple in the centre (see *Warts and verrucas*).

LARGE ROUND FLAT SPOTS WITH A CIRCULAR RING IN THE CENTRE look a little like targets, and in fact are knows as **target lesions**.

They are a sign of **erythema multiforme**, which is usually a reaction to an infection or drugs. The spots generally appear on the hands, feet, arms and legs.

Usually, no treatment is necessary, but CHECK WITH YOUR DOCTOR to confirm the diagnosis and identify the cause.

BLISTERING AROUND THE CHILD'S LIPS at the same time as erythema multiforme, is a more serious sign and should be CHECKED BY A DOCTOR STRAIGHT AWAY.

SPOTS IN A RING AROUND THE CHILD'S MOUTH AND THE BRIDGE OF THE NOSE are sometimes a sign of solvent abuse (see *Reading and school problems*).

SQUINT

Medically speaking, a squint (or cast) means that the child's eyes are pointing in different directions; it has nothing to do with screwing up his or her eyelids. Around one in fifteen children have a squint to some degree.

A SQUINT is normal in babies up to the age of about six weeks. After this age, the eyes should both point straight towards whatever the child is looking at. Some babies and young children have an **occasional squint**, when one eye will turn away from time to time if the child is very tired. This kind of squint almost always clears on its own with time, though if you notice it once a day or more, then CHECK WITH YOUR DOCTOR.

Normally the brain puts together the images from the two eyes to form a single three-dimensional picture. But if the child has a squint and the two eyes are looking in different directions, even slightly different, the picture will be blurred and the brain won't be able to make sense of it.

The way the child's brain copes with this problem is to ignore the image from one eye. Although both eyes are working fine, the child is actually only perceiving the image from one eye. He or she can see clearly, although only in two dimensions.

The problem is that eventually the brain will permanently ignore the image from the squinting eye. The eye becomes, in effect, totally blind and is called a **lazy eye**. This is a danger in a squint that hasn't been treated before the age of six or eight years, and is virtually inevitable after the age of ten years.

This is why spotting a squint, and treating it in time, is so important. Checking for a squint forms an important part of the routine checks that all babies and young children are offered, regularly, up to the age of about five years.

GUIDANCE

Spotting a squint in your child may be straightforward, or may be very difficult. If the squint is severe then it should be quite obvious, with the two eyes clearly pointing in different directions. But be cautious when checking small babies; often they have a very wide bridge to their nose, giving the impression that they are cross eyed when in fact they aren't.

❖   ❖   ❖

A better guide is to check the light reflection. If you look at your child's eyes, you will see the reflection of the window or electric light in his or her iris (the coloured area of the eye). If you can't then turn him or her until you can. Check the position of this tiny reflection in each eye. If the eyes are straight, the reflection should be in the same position in each eye. If the reflections are in different position, then CHECK WITH YOUR DOCTOR as this raises the possibility of a squint, although it may also be normal.

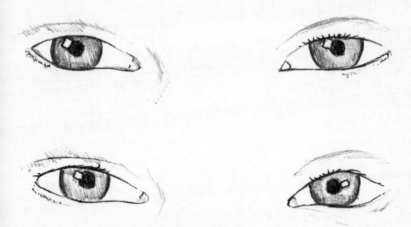

Squint; the light reflection is unequal

DOCTOR'S TREATMENT
SEE YOUR DOCTOR if you have any suspicion that your
child may have a squint.

❖   ❖   ❖

Treatment of a squint depends on the cause. Sometimes the
problem is that one eye isn't seeing properly in the first
place, and the child needs to wear glasses. Otherwise,
covering the good eye with a patch – to force the squinting
eye to straighten – usually works, although the child may
have to wear the patch for many months.

❖   ❖   ❖

Nowadays surgeons often prefer to correct the squint by
surgery while the child is still a toddler.

THROAT, SORE

The term sore throat covers a wide range of possibilities from minor discomfort on swallowing, to an ill child with a high temperature, shivers, sweats and vomiting.

TONSILLITIS is one form of sore throat in which the tonsils, the two fleshy glands at the back of the throat, are inflamed and infected. It is most common in children up to the age of about eight years old. After this, the tonsils usually start to shrink.

If your child is old enough to open his or her mouth wide, stick out the tongue and say 'aaah', then you will be able to see the tonsils as red swellings at the back of the throat, one on either side of the **uvula** (the 'bell clapper' that dangles down in the middle of the throat).

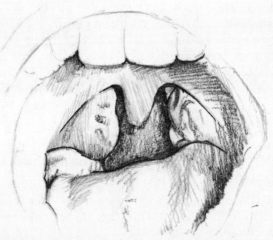

*You can see the tonsils as red swellings
at the back of your child's throat*

Swollen tonsils don't mean much – many children with repeated colds and sore throats have permanently huge tonsils. Very red tonsils with flecks of white or yellow pus on them are more likely to suggest tonsillitis.

In fact, whether a sore throat is caused by tonsillitis, or simply by infection of the other glands and tissues in the throat, isn't very important. Its effect on your child, and his or her overall degree of illness and discomfort, is much more significant.

SYMPTOMS OF A SORE THROAT may be, in fact, nothing more than that the throat is sore or scratchy, especially on swallowing. Older children may have a cough and cold too, and younger children may have signs of croup (see *Breathing, noisy or difficult*).

The pain usually starts suddenly, often with a temperature. This may be mild, or there may be a severe fever, with the risk of febrile fits in susceptible children (see *Fits*). A high temperature may produce shivers and sweats.

Pains in the abdomen are common, due to swelling of glands inside the abdomen (see *Pain in the abdomen, sudden*). Glands in the neck may also be very swollen, and sometimes tender. Some children vomit, usually no more than two or three times, and most will lose their appetite. Earaches are common, usually caused by the sore throat, but they should be CHECKED BY THE DOCTOR in case the child has an ear infection, too (see *Pain or discharge in the ear*).

Severely affected children will seem quite ill in general, tired and weak and often dizzy, too. A rash over the body together with flushed cheeks suggests scarlet fever (see *Rashes, sudden*).

Usually the symptoms start to improve after four to seven days, although a severe sore throat may take many more days to clear.

CAUSE OF SORE THROATS. Around three-quarters are caused by **viruses**, and there is no treatment which will make these better more quickly. The remaining one-quarter are caused by **bacteria**, usually by a bacterium known as **haemolytic streptococcus**. Antibiotic treatment would probably shorten this kind of sore throat by a day or two, although no one is precisely sure of the extent of the benefit.

DOCTOR'S TREATMENT
The problem is that it isn't possible from looking at the throat, or from checking the child's symptoms, to know whether a sore throat is caused by a bacterium or a virus.

A throat swab sent to a hospital laboratory for analysis will give an answer, but in most cases your GP will have to wait for up to a week for the result – by which time your child's throat is likely to have improved, anyway.

❖   ❖   ❖

This has led to **different opinions on the best treatment for sore throats**.

Some doctors reason that, since antibiotics may help about one-quarter of cases to get better more quickly, they should be given to everyone with a sore throat.

Some take the opposite point of view. They point out that antibiotic treatment inevitably carries the risk of side effects, such as thrush infection, diarrhoea and skin rashes, as well as the very tiny danger of dangerous or even fatal reactions. They say that since antibiotics aren't going to help most people with a sore throat, and as the benefits aren't certain anyway, they are best avoided.

❖   ❖   ❖

In fact, most doctors fall somewhere between these two extremes, and may suggest trying antibiotics for a child who is generally unwell, or in a considerable amount of pain or distress.

COMPLICATIONS, that is, other problems that are set off by the sore throat, are very rare. Rheumatic fever (damage to the heart muscle) and nephritis (kidney damage) used to be risks after a sore throat caused by a bacterial infection, but they are very rare indeed nowadays.

A **quinsy** is an abscess around the tonsil; besides severe throat pain and difficulty swallowing his or her own saliva, the child will have a large swelling on one side of the throat. SEE A DOCTOR if you suspect a quinsy, as treatment with antibiotics or surgery is necessary.

LOSING THE VOICE is common with, or sometimes without, a sore throat and suggests **laryngitis** – meaning that the infection has travelled down to reach the child's larynx (voice box). Complete rest of the voice (not even whispering – this puts a strain on the vocal chords too) and inhaling steam, are the best treatment. SEE YOUR DOCTOR if your child's voice doesn't return within a few days.

HOME TREATMENT
Treatment for a sore throat really means treating the symptoms until they get better on their own. Give paracetamol (see dosage, page 11) for pain and fever, and encourage your child to drink as much as possible – cool drinks are usually best.

❖　　❖　　❖

Inhaling steam over a bowl of steaming water sometimes helps, but be careful to avoid scalds.

❖　　❖　　❖

Older children may find relief from gargling with salt water. Children over 12 years old may gargle with soluble asprin, which is more helpful.

❖　　❖　　❖

Antiseptic or anaesthetic sprays and lozenges from the chemist may help the symptoms, although they won't clear the throat any more quickly and may, themselves, start to inflame the throat if used for longer than a few days.

❖   ❖   ❖   ❖   ❖

GUIDANCE
SEE YOUR DOCTOR if your child

❖ has a sore throat and is generally ill (see *Ill – should your child see the doctor?*), OR

❖ isn't able to keep liquids down, OR

❖ isn't able to swallow his or her own saliva (this suggests a possibly serious blockage such as quinsy or epiglottitis – see *Breathing, noisy or difficult*) OR

❖ makes a hoarse noise on breathing in (possible croup or epiglottitis – see *Breathing, noisy or difficult*).

❖   ❖   ❖

SEE A DOCTOR if the sore throat persists for more than ten days (possibility of an infection such as glandular fever).

TIREDNESS

SUDDEN TIREDNESS is very common and usually means that the child has developed, or has started to come down with, an infection such as a cold, flu or sore throat. Usually the child gradually picks up as the infection disappears, but some infections can leave a child shattered for weeks afterwards.

Several **virus infections** can do this although the most notorious is **glandular fever**; usually this starts as a sore throat. The tiredness generally improves after weeks or months (see **Long-term tiredness**, below).

Sudden tiredness in a child who is thirsty, drinking and peeing more than usual and possibly with abdominal pain and loss of weight may suggest **diabetes** and should be CHECKED BY A DOCTOR IMMEDIATELY.

LONG-TERM TIREDNESS persisting for more than a couple of weeks, may be due to the aftermath of a virus infection (see above). Usually there is no treatment apart from encouraging your child to do as much as he or she can, and waiting for a few weeks or, rarely, months.

Emotional problems affect children as well as adults and may cause a variety of symptoms, including tiredness. The child may be anxious, have trouble sleeping, be unkeen to go to school or show other signs of distress. Lack of sleep, by itself, is probably a rare cause of tiredness, but may be a problem if the child isn't sleeping or goes to bed very late (see *Sleep problems*).

Tiredness may be quite normal at some ages, depending upon what the parents expect. Pre-school children may have bursts of energetic activity but they often tire easily and may spend quite long periods exhausted, too. Energetic children sometimes seem to slow right down as soon as they reach puberty, and again this seems to be quite natural.

Some drugs may cause drowsiness or tiredness, and you should CHECK WITH YOUR DOCTOR about any your child is taking.

Anaemia, a shortage of red cells in the blood, does occur in children although it isn't often severe enough to cause tiredness; SEE YOUR DOCTOR, who can spot it with a blood test (see *Paleness*).

Long-term infections that haven't been spotted, may cause no symptoms apart from tiredness and, sometimes, retarded growth. Kidney infections and chest infections, such as tuberculosis, are possible causes.

❖   ❖   ❖   ❖   ❖

GUIDANCE
SEE YOUR DOCTOR if your child

❖   is tired and the red membrane, revealed by pulling down the lower eyelid, is pale (possibility of anaemia – see *Paleness*), OR

❖   has other symptoms such as fever, shortage of breath, loss of appetite or poor weight gain, OR

❖   seems unusually tired and easily exhausted compared to other children of the same age.

An examination and possibly a blood test by the doctor may be all that is required, although rarely other tests will be necessary.

URINE
SYMPTOMS

Symptoms involving the urine are important because of the possibility of a **urine infection**, which should always be taken seriously in children. However, urinary symptoms don't always mean an infection.

PASSING MORE WATER THAN USUAL may, rarely, be a symptom of **diabetes**. The child will be thirsty, drink more than normal, and may be tired and lose weight. SEE A DOCTOR IMMEDIATELY if diabetes is even remotely possible.

More commonly, a cold or other infection, or drinking more than usual – which may become a habit and sometimes suggests an emotional problem – is the cause.

Very rarely, kidney damage is to blame.

PAIN ON PASSING WATER may indicate a urine infection, although sometimes it simply means that there is an irritation around the end of the **urethra**, the tube leading from the bladder through which the child urinates. This could be caused by **balanitis** in a boy (an infection under the foreskin – see *Foreskin problems*) or **vulvitis** in a girl (an infection around the vagina – see *Vagina, sore or discharging*).

URINE INFECTIONS may cause no symptoms at all. More often the child will experience pain in the urethra (see above) on passing water, and may feel the urge to pass small amounts of water very often. Younger children may lose their ability to be dry, and suddenly start to wet the bed at night or their pants by day. The urine may appear cloudy and smelly, although this by itself doesn't prove that an infection is present. The child may have a temperature, which may be slightly or very high. Sometimes a child will be quite severely ill with a high temperature, vomiting, sweats and shivers.

Any combination of these symptoms may be present in any degree of severity, and if your child has any of them you should CHECK WITH YOUR DOCTOR.

Sometimes urine infections don't produce any obvious symptoms except for general tiredness, poor growth and slow weight gain (see *Tiredness*).

DOCTOR'S TREATMENT
The reason for taking urine infections so seriously in children is that they carry a **significant risk of permanent kidney damage**. Girls are much more prone to infection than boys, and up to two per cent probably have one at some time in their childhood. Around ten per cent of these may be left with kidney damage.

❖　　　❖　　　❖

Treatment of a urine infection is with a course of antibiotics in the first place, to prevent kidney scarring. Your doctor will try at all costs to send a urine sample to the hospital laboratory first, as it is so important to be sure of the diagnosis.

❖　　　❖　　　❖

Further tests may then follow, to see if there is any reason why your child has developed the infection. The tests themselves will depend on the age of your child.

Permanent kidney damage is very unlikely after the age of about six years, although you should still CHECK WITH YOUR DOCTOR if you suspect an infection. It is most likely under the age of four years. So, as a general rule, the younger the child the greater the risk of damage and the more tests are likely to be needed to check that all is well.

❖   ❖   ❖

Sometimes the tests show that urine is leaking back from the bladder into the **ureters** (the tubes connecting the kidneys to the bladder). This makes the child prone to urine infections, but usually corrects itself in time. Occasionally surgery is necessary.

❖   ❖   ❖

Sometimes the problem is with the kidneys themselves, which are scarred or deformed. Some children who are prone to recurrent infections may need to take antibiotics every day as a preventative measure, until they grow out of their tendency to infections.

❖   ❖   ❖   ❖   ❖

GUIDANCE
SEE YOUR DOCTOR if your child has any of the symptoms mentioned above which suggest a urinary infection.

❖   ❖   ❖

If you can take a sample of your child's urine to the surgery in a clean jar (washed out with boiled water, not soap or disinfectant), this could be very helpful.

VAGINA, SORE OR DISCHARGING

A discharging or sore vagina is surprisingly common even in very young girls, and doesn't usually suggest a serious problem.

A VAGINAL DISCHARGE IN NEWBORN BABIES is quite normal in the first few days after birth. Usually the discharge is thin, white and watery, although there may be some bleeding after about a week. The cause is simply that the baby girl's vagina and womb is responding to the hormone oestrogen, from her mother, which is still in the baby's bloodstream.

A DISCHARGE AROUND PUBERTY is also common, as the vagina responds to the oestrogen hormone that the girl is now starting to produce for herself. The discharge is usually thin and white.

A DISCHARGE OR SORENESS AROUND THE VAGINA BETWEEN THESE TWO AGES is usually the result of small particles of dust, dirt, dead skin or faeces making their way into the entrance of the vagina. This sets off a mild superficial infection in the area, and the skin may become quite red and sore. This is **vulvitis**, an inflammation of the vulva (the skin around the outside of the girl's vagina).

Usually, the discharge is clear, and white or pale yellow in colour, although sometimes it may seem sticky or a little smelly. Some girls with sensitive skin seem to react badly to soap or bath bubbles, which may make the problem worse.

This is a very common problem and doesn't mean that your child is dirty or not properly cared for. Sometimes little girls' own hygiene in that area leaves something to be desired.

HOME TREATMENT
Treatment is usually simply a matter of doing the right things until the problem solves itself. Avoid soap or bubbles in the bath, but clean around your little girl's vagina with water every day.

❖   ❖   ❖

Clean only the bits you can see, it is fine to gently part the lips of her vagina to wipe the entrance, but don't try to put anything inside.

❖   ❖   ❖

Always wipe her bottom from front to back after she has been to the loo, to avoid wiping traces of faeces from her bottom towards her vagina. If she is old enough to do this for herself, make sure that she is wiping in the right direction.

❖   ❖   ❖

Cotton knickers are probably best; indoors it is a good idea to let her spend some time without anything on her bottom at all, if possible.

❖   ❖   ❖

A barrier cream, such as zinc and castor oil, may help protect the skin around this area.

A VERY ITCHY VAGINA usually with an itchy bottom too, which is worse at night, raises the possibility of **threadworms** (see *Itching anus*).

A LARGE AMOUNT OF DISCHARGE which may be thick and dark yellow or brown in colour, may suggest a foreign object in the vagina (see *Foreign objects*). The discharge may be bloodstained, and sometimes very smelly.

SEXUAL ABUSE may cause infections and discharge, although this isn't a common cause and certainly nobody will start jumping to conclusions simply because your daughter has a discharge.

A RED SORE AREA around the vagina in baby girls who are still in nappies, may be the start of nappy rash (see *Nappy rash*).

❖   ❖   ❖   ❖   ❖

GUIDANCE
SEE YOUR DOCTOR if

◆   your daughter has a discharge which persists after three weeks despite the measures mentioned above, OR

◆   the discharge is thick, smelly or in large amounts (possibility of a foreign object, or a more serious infection), OR

◆   the skin around is very itchy (possibility of thread-worms), or red and sore (may be infected).

VOMITING

Vomiting is a common symptom in children, and there are a large number of possible causes. In some ways, more important than the cause of the vomiting is to know how severely it is affecting your child.

VOMITING IN BABIES may be due to possetting or rumination. This isn't actually vomiting, and is normal and quite harmless (see *Feeding problems in babies*).

Other feeding problems can cause vomiting too. Rarer causes include **intussusception**, a blockage of the bowel (see *Blood in the stools*), travel sickness and the side effects of drugs.

VOMITING IN CHILDREN OF ANY AGE, which appears suddenly, is usually due to an infection. This may be **gastroenteritis**, an infection of part of the bowel itself (see below), although almost any infection which makes the child generally unwell – a sore throat or ear, urine or chest infection – can cause vomiting. The child will usually have a temperature also.

VOMITING WITH A HEADACHE in a child who has a temperature or is generally unwell, is also likely to be caused by an infection, such as flu or a sore throat. It should be taken seriously, however, as it raises the possibility of **meningitis** (see *Neck, stiff or painful*).

VOMITING WITH PAIN IN THE ABDOMEN is common, since **gastroenteritis** often causes cramping pains that come and go, usually in the upper part of the abdomen or in the lower part to one side.

Repeated vomiting and retching may itself be painful, as it can cause a strain of the muscles in the upper part of the abdomen. However, check for the pattern of pain that would suggest more serious problems, such as **appendicitis** (see *Pain in the abdomen, sudden*).

EXCITEMENT, ANXIETY OR TRAVEL SICKNESS sometimes cause vomiting in susceptible children.

SWALLOWING POISON may produce vomiting, which is also a side effect of many drugs (see *Poisoning*).

BLOOD IN THE VOMIT is actually quite common, especially in older children, with repeated retching and vomiting due to **gastroenteritis** (see below).

Usually the cause is a tear in the lining of the stomach, the result of repeated straining of the stomach muscles. Although it looks dramatic, the blood loss isn't dangerous, and usually soon settles, although it should be CHECKED BY A DOCTOR to rule out much rarer causes, such as a stomach ulcer.

Sometimes blood from a nosebleed will trickle down into the stomach, to reappear as dark brown bloodstained vomit some time later.

GASTROENTERITIS means a stomach bug. In fact, the infection may affect the stomach and upper part of the bowel to produce mainly vomiting, or the lower part of the bowel to produce mainly diarrhoea and cramping pains, or a combination of the two.

The vomiting is usually quite severe; it appears suddenly and the poor child may vomit several times an hour, retching even when his or her stomach is empty. Mostly, the diarrhoea is watery but may occasionally be bloody (see *Diarrhoea*). Usually the child has a temperature and may feel generally achy and fluish.

Gastroenteritis is infectious and several members of the family may be affected at once, particularly children. Usually the cause is a **virus infection**, although sometimes **bacterial food poisoning** is to blame. The symptoms may be identical whether your child caught the infection from someone else or from something he or she ate, and often it isn't possible to pin-point the source.

Generally, the vomiting in gastroenteritis settles within 24 or 48 hours, although the diarrhoea and stomach cramps may carry on for several days longer.

HOME TREATMENT
Treatment of gastroenteritis means keeping your child comfortable and drinking as much as possible to avoid the risk of **dehydration** (see below). Except in certain unusual forms of food poisoning, there is no treatment which will clear the symptoms any more quickly.

❖   ❖   ❖

Paracetamol (see dosage, page 11) is useful for fever and pain. Anti-sickness drugs don't generally work for this kind of illness, and some may have side effects in young children. They are generally best avoided.

❖   ❖   ❖

It is probably best to keep your child off milk, as this is difficult to digest, and may make diarrhoea worse. Even young babies will take no harm through not having milk for a few days.

❖   ❖   ❖

Drinking some form of fluid is vital; juice, or plain water, may be fine for older children.

❖   ❖   ❖

Babies and young children should have a salt/sugar mixture, available as a powder from the chemist to mix with water. This is designed to be easily absorbed and to replace the fluid and salt lost through vomiting.

Don't try to mix salt and sugar yourself as a slight mistake with the proportions may make matters worse rather than better. If you don't have the powder to hand, then use water or juice in the meantime.

❖   ❖   ❖

Give frequent sips every few minutes rather than a big drink all at once, as this is simply likely to come straight back up again. Liquid at room temperature is less likely to upset the stomach than hot or cold drinks.

DEHYDRATION is the biggest danger with vomiting, and to a lesser extent with diarrhoea or excessive urine production (in diseases such as diabetes). Dehydration means a loss of body fluids, although the loss of salt and other chemicals that accompany the fluid loss is potentially dangerous too.

Because of the risk of dehydration, **gastroenteritis is the fifth commonest killer of babies in this country** and an even more important problem world wide. It is vital to watch for, and be able to recognise, the signs of dehydration.

GUIDANCE
The first sign of dehydration is a dry mouth. Simply wash your hands and place a finger inside your child's mouth to check whether the mouth and tongue feel dry.

The child will usually start to produce less urine too.

❖   ❖   ❖

These signs suggest that the child has lost up to about five per cent of his or her body fluid. This may not be a serious loss, especially in older children, but should nevertheless be CHECKED BY A DOCTOR.

❖   ❖   ❖

Signs of more serious fluid loss include sunken eyes and, in babies, a sunken fontanelle (the soft spot on the top of the head). The child's skin starts to lose elasticity.

Pinch the skin on the back of your child's hand or over the abdomen between your fingers and thumb; normally the fold of skin springs back immediately once you let go. With

261

dehydration the skin sinks slowly back into shape, and may feel more doughy than normal.

❖   ❖   ❖

These signs suggest that the child has lost between five and ten per cent of body fluid, and should be SEEN BY A DOCTOR IMMEDIATELY.

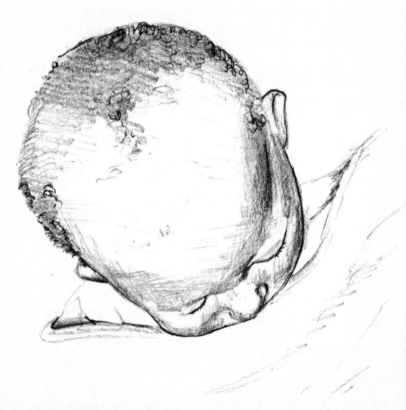

A dry mouth is the first sign of dehydration. More serious signs include sunken eyes and fontanelle, doughy skin and eventually drowsiness and collapse

❖   ❖   ❖

As **dehydration becomes more severe**, the child becomes increasingly unwell with a rapid pulse, rapid breathing, pale mottled skin, and drowsiness which may progress into coma. This state is a MEDICAL EMERGENCY.

❖   ❖   ❖   ❖   ❖

SEE YOUR DOCTOR if your child

- is vomiting and has any signs of dehydration, OR

- has severe abdominal pain, OR

- has vomiting which doesn't settle in 24 hours (babies and toddlers), or 36 hours (older children), OR

- has bloodstained vomit, OR

- vomits after a head injury (see *Head injuries*), OR

- has signs suggesting meningitis (see *Neck, stiff or painful*), OR

- appears ill (see *Ill – should your child see the doctor?*).

WARTS AND VERRUCAS

Warts are caused by a skin infection with a virus called **human papilloma virus**. A verruca is simply a wart which is situated on the sole of the child's foot. Similar spots, called **molluscum contagiosum**, are caused by a different virus.

A WART first appears as a small skin-coloured lump. Some warts, called **plane warts**, tend to affect the hands and face and stay as small raised lumps with a flat top. More often, the wart develops a hard irregular surface, and may gradually grow larger. Often, several warts appear together in the same area.

Warts are completely harmless, and rarely cause any problems apart from teasing from the child's friends because his or her warts look ugly.

Although not highly infectious, they can be passed on by direct contact from one person to the other, or occasionally from changing room or shower room floors. It is possible for a child with a wart to spread it to another part of his or her own body.

VERRUCAS are simply warts on the soles of the feet. Like other warts they are harmless, although if they occur on an area of the foot that bears the child's weight (usually the heel, or the ball of the foot) they may cause pain on walking, as pressure from the child's weight forces the verruca into the skin.

Unlike other warts, verrucas don't grow out from the skin but are almost flat. They have a rough, slightly dark surface surrounded by a ring of hard, dead skin. Sometimes, the centre of the verruca contains tiny black dots; these are tiny blood clots inside the verruca.

HOME TREATMENT
Treatment of warts and verrucas often isn't necessary as they always disappear on their own, although this may take months or even years. On average, about half have disappeared after one year and most by 18 months, although a few take longer still.

❖   ❖   ❖

Warts that are particularly ugly and distressing to the child, or verrucas that cause pain on walking, may sometimes need treatment. Although there are several different forms of treatment, unfortunately none is guaranteed to do the trick.

❖   ❖   ❖

Wart creams and paints from the chemist are mostly designed to remove the layer of hard, dead skin over the wart or verruca and expose its core. They can burn normal skin, and you should protect the skin around the wart or verruca by smearing it with petroleum jelly.

They often take several weeks to have an effect. Most are designed to be applied a couple of times a week, but you should follow the instructions with the preparation you are using, and apply it less frequently if the surrounding skin becomes red or painful.

❖   ❖   ❖

Never apply any wart preparation to your child's face except on your doctor's advice, as these preparations are generally far too strong. In fact, many doctors prefer not to treat warts on the face at all. When a wart heals on its own, it does so without leaving a scar, whereas treatment often carries the risk of some scarring.

❖   ❖   ❖

For verrucas and hard, horny warts, it helps to soak the affected part in warm water every day and gently rub the dead skin away with a pumice stone or emery board.

DOCTOR'S TREATMENT
If home treatment doesn't work, SEE YOUR DOCTOR, who may be able to arrange for the wart or verruca to be destroyed by freezing, cutting or burning.

All of these methods can be painful and carry some risk of scarring, and several attempts may be necessary before the wart is finally destroyed. For these reasons many doctors won't apply them to young children.

PREVENTION
Prevention of **warts and verrucas** is difficult. Some swimming pools have rules banning children with verrucas. Certainly, wet pool sides and changing room floors can spread the infection, but many children have verrucas without knowing it and children with warts on their hands or elsewhere are just as likely to spread the virus. Nowadays, many experts say that it is simpler just to accept the risk of catching a harmless verruca.

❖   ❖   ❖

If your child has a verruca, and your local pool does insist on keeping out children with verrucas, then your child should wear a **plastic verruca sock**, available from the chemist, to the pool. This will cut out the risk of him or her spreading the virus.

MOLLUSCUM CONTAGIOSUM are small, round, raised, shiny pink spots that usually have a tiny dimple in the centre. They slowly grow, but don't usually become bigger than about half a centimetre across.

As with warts, they often appear in crops, and several may appear in different parts of the body at once. They aren't painful or itchy, although children with sensitive skin may develop sore red patches of inflamed skin around them.

They are caused by a **skin infection with pox virus**, different from the virus which causes warts. As with warts, they disappear on their own with time, usually within a year or so. The spots are infectious, and often several members of the family are affected at the same time.

HOME TREATMENT

Treatment of **molluscum**, as with warts, often isn't necessary. If you do feel that your child needs treatment, then the treatment for warts (see above) may work well.

DOCTOR'S TREATMENT

The doctor can destroy the spots by squeezing them with forceps, or injecting them with a poisonous chemical such as phenol.

However, these measures can be painful, and may frighten small children.

WEIGHT PROBLEMS

Weight is one of the few ready measures of a child's state of health. Babies who don't seem to be gaining weight as they should are a common cause of distress and anxiety, even though most turn out fine in the end. Older children who seem too skinny, who lose weight, or who are overweight, also cause worry – which fortunately often turns out to be needless in the end.

DISCOVERING WHETHER YOUR CHILD IS GROWING AT THE RIGHT RATE isn't always easy. Different babies and children grow at different rates, and the only way to be sure that yours is gaining weight at the rate that is right for him or her is to plot the weight on a **centile chart**.

USING A CENTILE CHART. When your child was born you were probably given a record book (the type varies around the country) which included centile charts for plotting his or her growth. There may be separate charts for weight, height and head size.

On the chart will be a line, **the 50th centile line**, which marks the average weight at any particular age. If you mark your child's weight on the chart, you can tell at a glance whether it is above average (above the 50th centile line) or below average (below this line) compared to other children of the same age.

But, marking one single weight reading on the chart isn't very informative. Some children will be above average weight, and some below, quite naturally. In order to tell if your child's weight gain is abnormal, you must mark his or her weight several times, at different ages, on the chart. Now you have several marks which can be joined to form a line.

As a general rule, if your child's weight line **runs parallel** to the 50th centile line – whether above or below it – then he or she is gaining weight properly. If it is **heading away from** the 50th centile line then there may be a problem which should be checked.

This is a simple explanation, and there is more to using centile charts than this. This is why doctors and health visitors are trained in their use, and will plot your baby's growth on a centile chart whenever you attend routine check-ups or baby clinics.

Older children aren't usually weighed and measured regularly, but your doctor or health visitor will still use a centile chart if you think there is a problem. For this reason it is helpful if you can take with you any weight or height records from the past, so they can also be plotted.

BABIES WHO AREN'T GAINING WEIGHT as they should, may turn out not to have a problem at all (see **Using a centile chart**, above). Otherwise there may be several causes.

Feeding problems, which can occur in bottle-fed or breast-fed babies, are the most likely cause in very young babies, and your health visitor is specifically trained to help (see *Feeding problems in babies*).

A slowing of weight gain for two or three weeks is common after an infection such as gastroenteritis, or an ear infection, but your baby's weight should bounce back afterwards. Much more rarely, infections such as chest or urine infections that don't clear, may cause long-term problems.

Some babies have disease affecting their bowel which prevents them from being able to absorb their food properly. YOU SHOULD SEE YOUR DOCTOR. **Cystic fibrosis** is one possibility. Another is **coeliac disease**, where the child can't tolerate wheat and rye and may develop diarrhoea, with poor weight gain, as soon as he or she starts taking solids.

Other causes are rarer, but may need to be checked for by your doctor.

OLDER CHILDREN WHO SEEM SKINNY are usually, in fact, quite healthy; they simply have a light build. Again, the centile chart is the best guide to whether there really is a problem (see above).

If the weight gain is less than it should be, then **cystic fibrosis** or **coeliac disease** are possible causes (see above), although any long-term infection or illness such as **asthma** or **kidney infection** may be to blame, so CHECK WITH YOUR DOCTOR.

CHILDREN WHO ARE ACTUALLY LOSING WEIGHT are usually suffering from an infection such as flu, sore throat, ear infection or pneumonia. **Gastroenteritis** is a particularly common culprit as children can lose weight through fluid loss (see **Gastroenteritis** in *Vomiting*). The weight should start to shoot back up once the child starts to recover. If not, then weight loss is a potentially serious sign that should be CHECKED BY A DOCTOR.

CHILDREN WHO ARE VERY OVERWEIGHT run the risk of being fat in adult life. The child's eating habits may not be entirely to blame – some children do seem more prone to fat than others – but sensible eating is the only real remedy. This doesn't have to mean a strict diet, but healthy food without too much fat or sugar at meal times and a firm hand on sweets or snacks in between. Your health visitor should be able to advise and help.

Gland or hormone problems are very rarely to blame for overweight, but CHECK WITH YOUR DOCTOR if your child is fat and short for his or her age. Most fat children are tall for their age; a short fat child raises the rare possibility of a gland disorder.

❖　　❖　　❖　　❖　　❖

GUIDANCE
SEE YOUR DOCTOR if your child

❖　isn't gaining weight as his or her centile chart suggests, OR

- has a low weight and is lethargic, or prone to other symptoms such as vomiting or fever (may suggest a long-term infection), OR

- has a low weight with persistent diarrhoea (may suggest he or she isn't absorbing food properly due to cystic fibrosis or coeliac disease), OR

- is actually losing weight (apart from the immediate affects of an infection), OR

- is overweight and short for his or her age.

SEE YOUR HEALTH VISITOR if you are unsure or concerned about your child's overall growth and development.

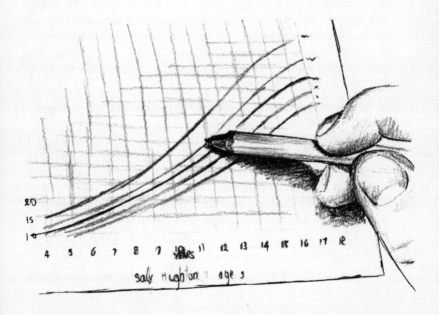

The only way to be sure that your child is gaining weight at the rate that is right for him or her is to plot the weight on a centile chart

271

WHEEZING

Wheezing is a high-pitched, almost musical sound which comes from the child's chest when he or she is breathing **out**.

Noise made by the child breathing **in** is not a wheeze, and has different causes (see *Breathing, noisy or difficult*).

Probably the only sound which could be confused with wheezing is phlegm bubbling in the child's throat during a cold. This doesn't sound as musical as a wheeze, usually occurs on breathing in as well as out, and may disappear temporarily after a cough.

WHEEZING IN BABIES AROUND THE AGE OF TWO TO SIX MONTHS is often a sign of **bronchiolitis**. This is a virus infection, usually with the same virus (**respiratory syncytial virus,** or **RSV**) that causes croup in older children and colds in adults. Some babies seem prone to this wheezy reaction to RSV infection.

At first the child develops a cold, but soon becomes wheezy and may start to breathe more quickly. The wheeze tends to be worse late at night. Often it is quite mild and doesn't distress the child, but occasionally it can cause severe and even dangerous difficulty in breathing. For this reason, SEE YOUR DOCTOR if your baby becomes wheezy. If he or she is wheezy and has any signs of difficulty in breathing (see *Breathing, noisy or difficult*) or is breathing increasingly quickly, then TAKE HIM OR HER TO CASUALTY IMMEDIATELY.

Most babies don't develop bronchiolitis more than once, but babies who have had it, do have a higher than normal chance of developing asthma later on.

ASTHMA is the most common and important cause of wheezing at all ages past six months. It affects around five per cent of children overall, and is becoming more common in this country.

Although wheezing is the most important characteristic of asthma, children who are mildly affected may not wheeze at all. Colds that always 'go on to the chest' and linger, or a persistent cough especially at night-time or after exercise, raise the possibility of asthma. More rarely, bad asthma that hasn't been diagnosed, may lead to stunted growth.

These symptoms usually come and go, and a child who is only mildly affected may seem fine in between times. **Exercise**, an **infection** such as a cold, or an **emotional shock**, may trigger an attack. Some children are affected by **allergy**, often to house dust or animals. They may only develop symptoms after they have visited friends who have pets.

Symptoms tend to be worse at night and first thing in the morning, and sometimes in the evening as well.

Eczema (see *Rashes, long-term*) and **hay fever** (see *Hay fever and nose allergies*), tend to be associated with asthma, and a child who suffers from one has a greater risk of suffering the others too. Some children with hay fever, an allergy to pollen in late spring, become wheezy at the same time.

Asthma usually improves after a period of around 10 to 20 years. Although there is no cure, it can usually be kept well under control with modern treatments.

❖   ❖   ❖   ❖   ❖

GUIDANCE
Treatment of asthma is a matter for close cooperation between you, your child, your doctor and possibly other people such as your doctor's practice nurse, a specialised asthma nurse, or a hospital clinic.

❖   ❖   ❖

More and more emphasis nowadays is being placed on **you and your child as key people** in this relationship. An asthmatic child's condition can vary wildly from day to day, and by doing the right things and making the right adjustments to his or her medication, you may be able to keep much better control over the asthma.

❖   ❖   ❖

Treatment needs to be PRESCRIBED BY, AND SUPERVISED BY, YOUR DOCTOR.

Inhalers, either taken regularly to prevent attacks or as necessary to treat symptoms, are the mainstay of treatment for most children. The child inhales a dose of drug as a mist or powder which acts immediately on the lungs. Special forms of inhaler, or devices which attach to the inhaler, are usable by some children from the age of one year.

Oral treatment may be necessary for younger children, or to treat severe attacks at any age.

SEE YOUR DOCTOR if you think your child

❖   is truly wheezing at any stage, OR

❖   has a cough at night that lasts for more than a couple of weeks, OR

❖   coughs or is breathless first thing in the morning, OR

❖   coughs after exercise, OR

❖   when exercising, has to stop before his or her friends because of shortness of breath, wheezing or coughing.

❖   ❖   ❖

If in doubt, it might pay you to keep a diary of your child's symptoms, recording what they are and when they occur, for a few weeks.

Although your doctor can examine your child's chest for wheeze and perform basic tests of his or her lung function, the diagnosis of asthma rests most importantly of all on your child's symptoms and their pattern. Sometimes the doctor might suggest confirming the diagnosis by trying asthma treatment to see if it works.

274

❖   ❖   ❖

If you are still in doubt then SEE YOUR DOCTOR ANYWAY. Asthma can affect a child's growth if it isn't treated, and even though the symptoms seem mild, you may be amazed at the new child you discover once they are properly treated.

CHEST INFECTIONS may cause wheezing in older children, although often this is merely an unmasking of the symptoms of **asthma**.

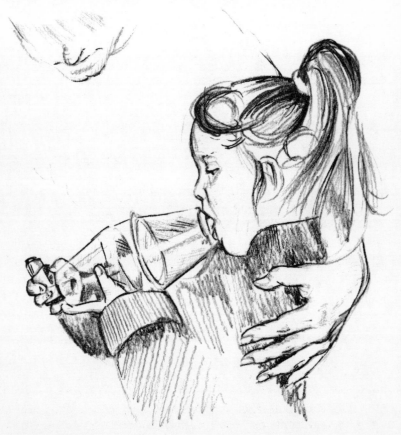

Young children may need special attachments to enable them to use an inhaler properly

INDEX

Section

Opening doors to the World of books

**Book Tokens
can be bought and
exchanged at most bookshops**